RECONSTRUCTIVE SURGERY
OF THE LONG BONES
WITH AUTOGENOUS AND HOMOGENOUS GRAFTS

from the Orthopaedic Department of the Wilhelmina Gasthuis,
University of Amsterdam (head: Prof. O. Verbeek M.D.)

RECONSTRUCTIVE SURGERY OF THE LONG BONES WITH AUTOGENOUS AND HOMOGENOUS GRAFTS

O. VERBEEK M.D. (Professor of Orthopaedics, University of Amsterdam),
M. J. KINGMA M.D. (Professor of Orthopaedics, University of Groningen)

with the collaboration of
A. VAN DEN HOOFF M.D. (Reader in Histology, University of Amsterdam),
R. STEENDIJK M.D. (Reader in Endocrinology, University of Amsterdam)

H. E. STENFERT KROESE N.V. / LEIDEN 1973

ISBN 978-94-011-9663-5   ISBN 978-94-011-9661-1 (eBook)
DOI 10.1007/978-94-011-9661-1
Library of Congress Catalogue Card Number 72-88777

CONTENTS

CHAPTER I

INTRODUCTION

After my appointment as head of the Orthopaedic Department in the Surgical Clinic of the Wilhelmina Gasthuis in Amsterdam, January 1953, I have had the privilege of a close and daily co-operation with my second-incharge M. J. Kingma. Amongst other problems, reconstructive surgery with the aid of bone-grafting captured the interest of both of us. In vol. XII, fasc. 3 (1960) of the Archivum Chirurgicum Neerlandicum Kingma wrote: 'The use of calf bone preserved by refrigeration was introduced into surgery in the Netherlands by Meiss in 1951. After the appearance of Meiss' reports on his favourable results, many other surgeons wished to employ this method and in order to cope with the numerous requests for material, a national bone transplantation service for calf bone was instituted in 1952 under the patronage of the Netherlands Red Cross with Kingma as its medical director'. In 1953 we considered *homogenous graft* to provide a better 'biological intermedium' than calf bone graft. Consequently we developed a bone-bank for homogenous grafts in our department from that date.

After 18 years of experience we have been able to demonstrate clinically and radiologically that in some cases a '*biological fixation*' can be maintained with the homogenous graft during the reconstruction by '*graduated*' function. Kingma controlled the results and arranged the data.

In this process of regeneration and consolidation the homogenous graft is assimilated into reconstruction of the original form by the penetrating blood vessels which accompany the deposition and reabsorption of bone.

To illustrate our results in this introductory chapter we herewith give some examples.

In children we have observed that in cases where there is a defect in the continuity of a long bone, a homogenous graft will be transformed into a normal cylindrical shaft. :

Patient E.V., girl, born 2–7–1951 (no. 3, chapter VI), see opposite page.

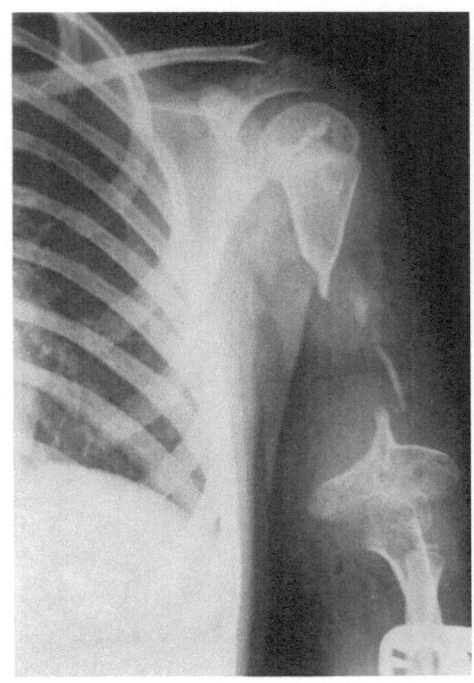

13-3-1957, defect-pseudarthrosis, right humerus

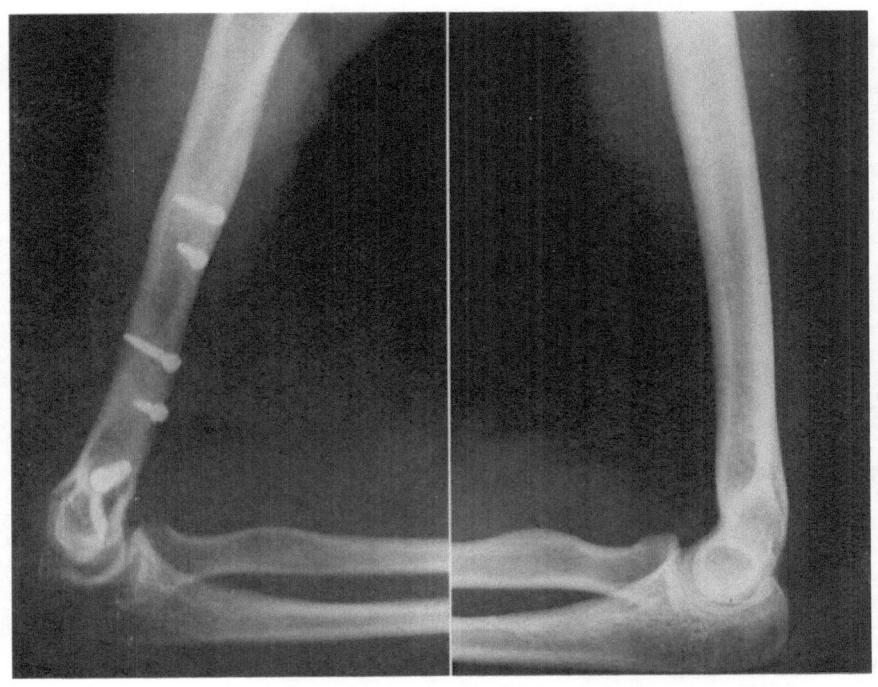

28-3-1967, satisfactory longitudinal growth of the humerus

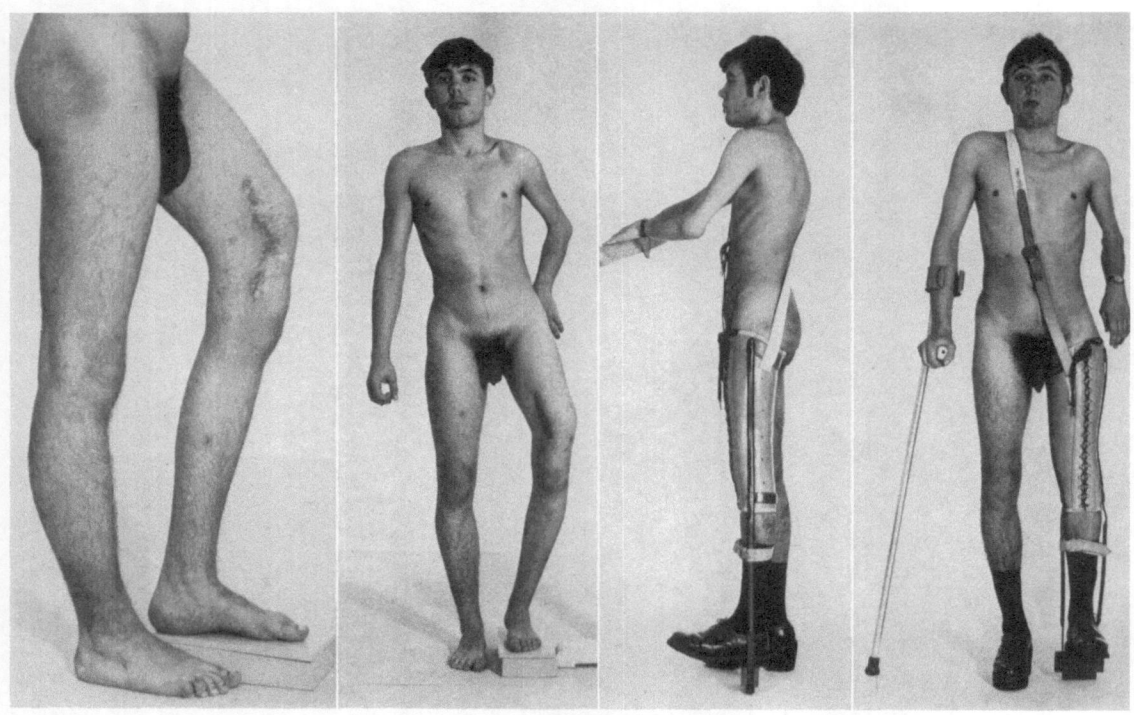

2–1–1967, pseudarthrosis after osteomyelitis   29–2–1968, 'after-treatment' in 'spring caliper'

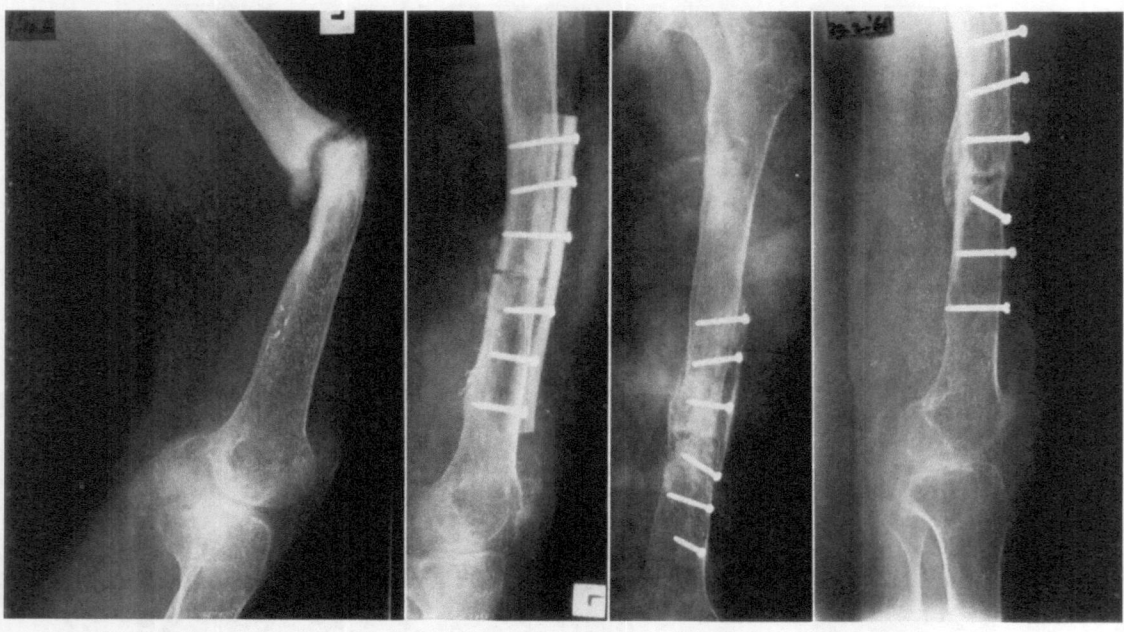

18–10–1966, pseudarthrosis after osteo-   3–1–1967,   19–1–1967   29–2–1968
myelitis as a newborn, left femur   osteosynthesis with
                                           homogenous graft

In children a pseudarthrosis caused by osteomyelitis can be completely healed by grafting:

Patient G.v.A., boy, born 12–6–1949

Treated in infancy because of septicaemia and osteomyelitis of the right femur. Pseudarthrosis of the left femur after a spontaneous fracture in October 1965.

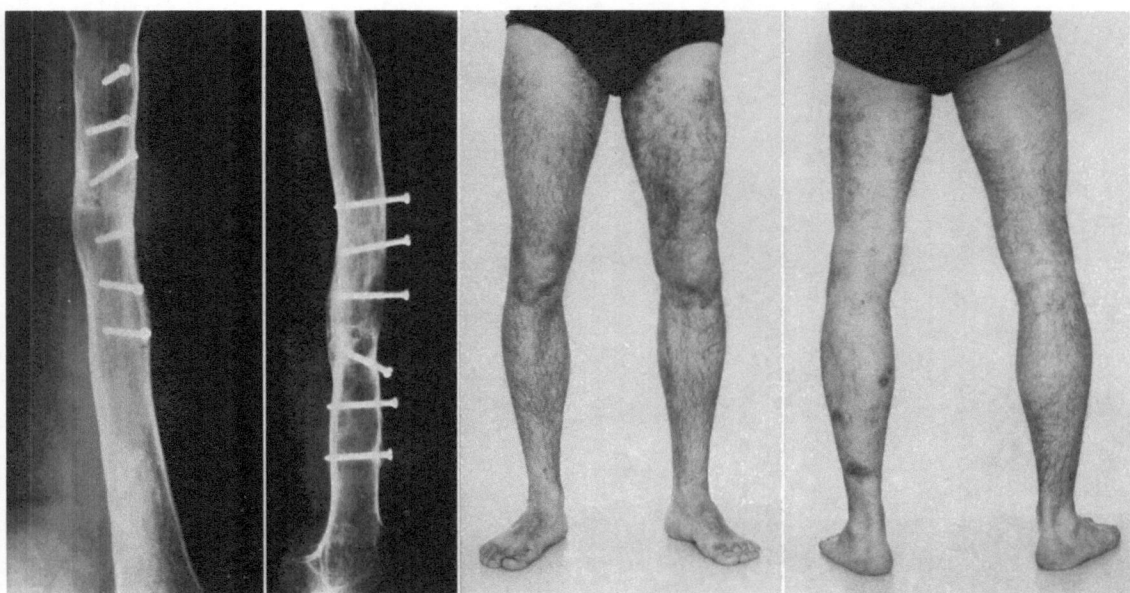

6–3–1969   6–3–1969

A particularly satisfactory result was observed in a case in which a Küntscher nail had been used to secure fixation of a spontaneous femoral fracture caused by metastasis of a hypernephroma. A homogenous graft was also applied to prevent rotation. The graft was completely assimilated in the reconstruction of the femur.

Patient C.M.R.B., female, born 4–11–1892

May 1948:   haematuria, on urological examination no abnormalities found; in the following years there was intermittent haematuria.

Sept. 1958:   pain along the distribution of the right sciatic nerve, later on colicky pains also.

Oct. 1959:   the same pain was present on the left side, pains on the right side had disappeared. On the X-ray a defect in the right wing of the sacrum was seen. Needle biopsy was negative; more X-rays, however, showed a cavity in the right femur.

Nov. 1959:   *spontaneous fracture* of the femur; osteosynthesis with Küntscher nail and homogenous graft. Path. anat. examination of material from the fracture site: no diagnosis possible. Results of investigations by physician could not explain the spontaneous fracture. On later X-rays the sacral defect had disappeared.

March 1963:   mild myocardial infarction.

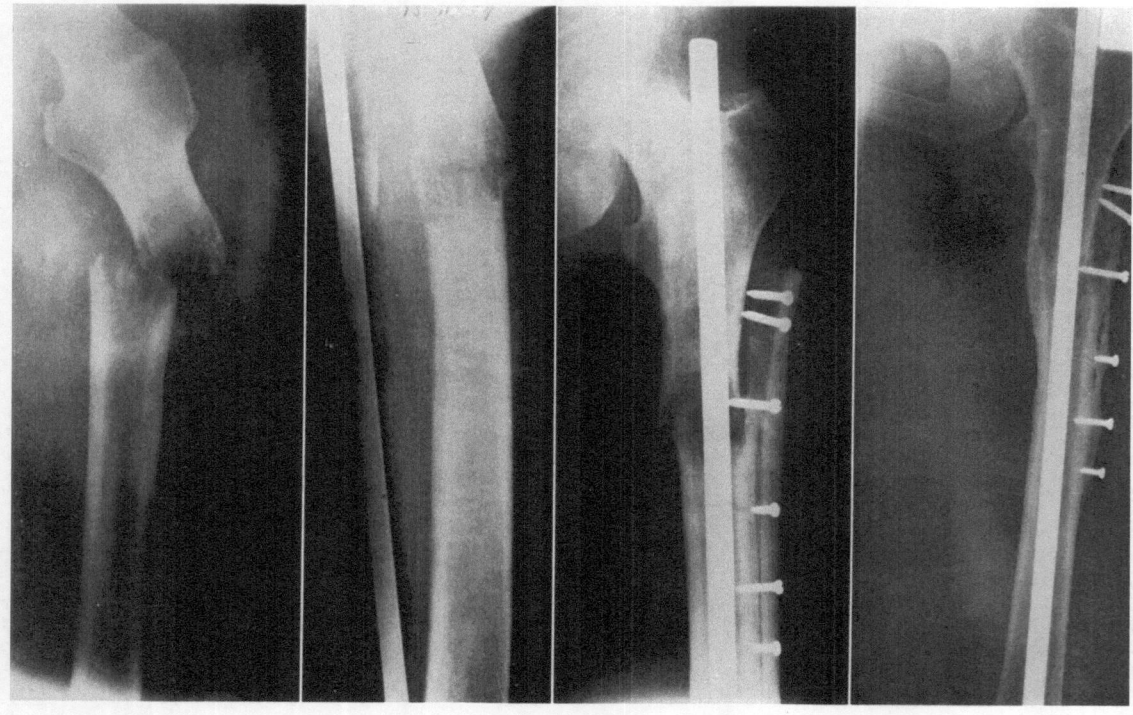

13–11–1959, metastasis hypernephroma, left femur   19–11–1959, osteosynthesis   22–1–1969, structural recon-
with Küntscher nail and   struction, normal function
homogenous graft

10

Sept. 1963:   patient noticed abdominal mass, which proved to be a kidney tumour. *Removal of the kidney concerned:* carcinoma of the Grawitz type.
Jan. 1969:   *structural reconstruction* of the femur with *normal* function. General condition normal.
Jan. 1972:   alive and well.

It is interesting to record that two years after the orthopaedic operation, the primary tumour was demonstrated elsewhere and removed. Up to now no recurrence has been observed. We will not attribute this to the homogenous graft, although we consider *immunological factors*.

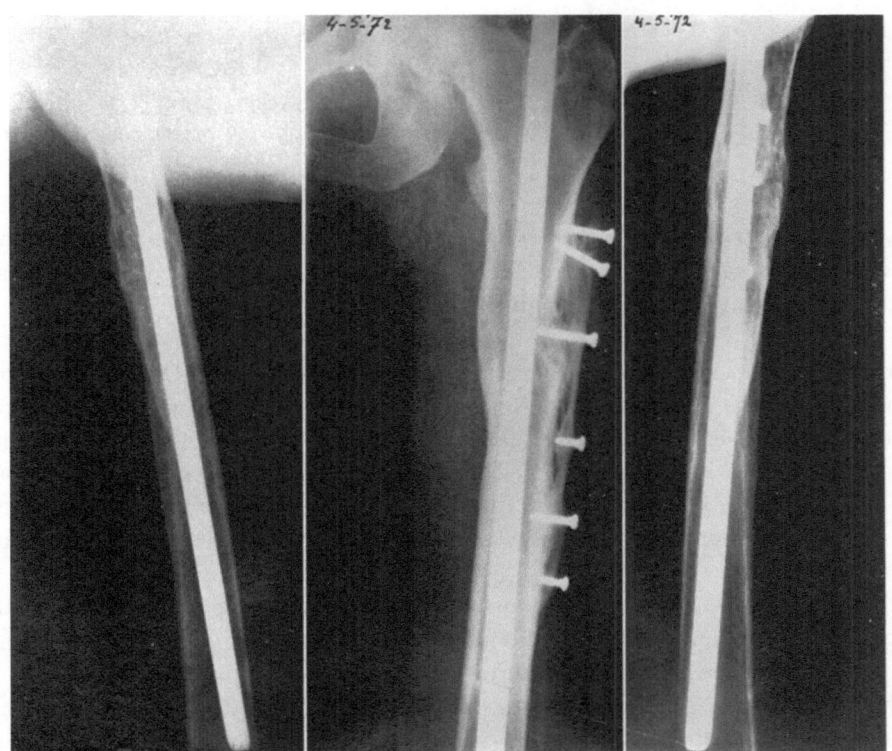

22–1–1969, structural recon-   4–5–1972, good condition
struction, normal function

In connection with the above, we refer to *patient J.V., male, born 7-1-1941 (no. 11, chapter V).* Sarcoma of the femur. X-ray therapy applied, followed by X-ray scarring of the skin, and pseudarthrosis of the femur. After satisfactory skin cover by plastic surgery we treated the pseudarthrosis by homogenous bone grafting. Lasting good result.

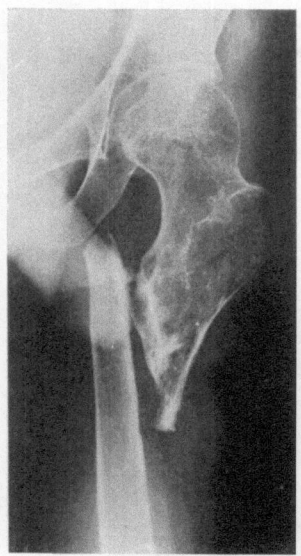 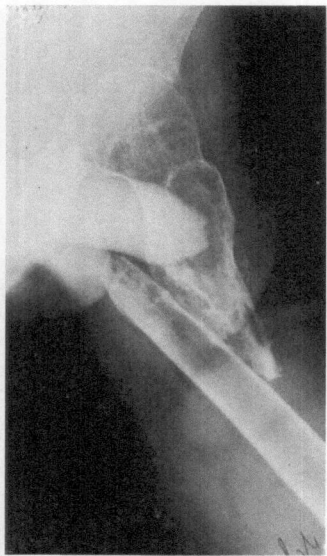 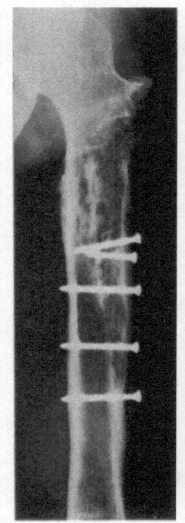 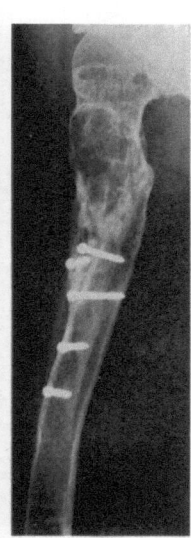

12-12-1957, pseudarthrosis of the left femur

19-4-1968, consolidated fracture, reconstruction of the shaft

After 15 years of experience we have gradually arrived at the indications for homogenous grafts used in reconstructive surgery of the skeletal system, and we are convinced that, serious disability can be prevented in many cases especially in children and elderly patients.

Concluding this introduction I would like to thank my co-author Prof. Dr. M. J. Kingma for the fruitful and harmonious co-operation during the years 1953-1969. Apart from his many clinical activities, he has performed particularly valuable work in the experimental laboratory of the Surgical Clinic, in collaboration with Prof. Dr. J. F. Hampe of the Pathological Anatomical Department of the Wilhelmina Gasthuis, and in particular for his co-operation in the clinical investigation into the usefulness of the homogenous graft in the *initial moulding* phase in orthopaedics and reconstructive surgery.
I also wish to thank Prof. Dr. D. B. Kroon for his hospitality in the Histological Institute, which created a close co-operation with his collaborateurs Dr. J. James, Dr. A. van den Hooff and Dr. R. Steendijk, to whom we have pleasure in acknowledging our appreciation.
I also wish to thank Prof. Dr. C. A. Wagenvoort and Prof. Dr. J. F. Hampe, of the Pathological Anatomical Department of the Wilhelmina Gasthuis and of the Pathological Department of the Antonie van Leeuwenhoekhuis, for their collaboration in developing the pathological and anatomical aspects of the clinical diseases of the musculo-skeletal system. These are often so difficult to interpret as regards their nature and prognosis.

Many thanks and appreciation are due to our former assistent Dr. K. Dey, who, notwithstanding his orthopaedic practice, has rendered the English translation of this work, which makes this publication more accessible.

I thank Mr. W. H. Camstra and his collaborators of the photographical laboratory of the Wilhelmina Gasthuis for the great dedication and skill with which they have reproduced the X-ray photographs. These photographs provide a real demonstration of our views on reconstructive processes in orthopaedics.

I have also pleasure in acknowledging our appreciation of the pleasant and sound co-operation with former and present assistants during the period 1953-1971.

A great amount of work in collecting data, discussing the composition and transmitting thoughts into typescript has been performed by our secretaries Miss A. M. Schaafsma and Miss S. D. Linschoten, to whom our sincere thanks and appreciation are due.

O. VERBEEK

CHAPTER II

THE BONE-BANK

Bone tissue for homo-transplantation can be obtained from the following sources:

1. *Operations*. This source does not yield much. The number of operations yielding bone tissue suitable for this purpose, is too small. Material from amputations performed because of trauma, infection, malignancy, circulatory disturbances with necrosis is not suitable. Also we dare not use ribs from thoracotomies performed for tumour or tuberculosis, apart from the fact that ribs are poor material for transplantation.
2. *Members of the patient's family*. In some cases we have obtained a graft from a parent on behalf of their children.
3. *Corpse*. This source yields a very good supply. Practically all our homo-transplantations have been performed with bone obtained from dead bodies.
   The corpse must comply with certain conditions. It must be the body of someone who died suddenly and has not been suffering from an infectious disease or malignancy. Age is of no importance. Most suitable are sudden cardiac deaths, or sudden deaths resulting from trauma, provided there is no injury of the skin.

We always ask for consent of the relatives, the medical superintendent of the hospital and if necessary, the public prosecutor. Observing all the routine of an aseptic operation, the iliac crests, the shafts of the femur and tibia are removed from the body, commencing within a few hours (maximum six hours) after death.

The material obtained is wrapped up still under sterile conditions and promptly placed in the deep-freeze. With the aid of wooden sticks and plaster the stability of the lower extremities is restored. Blood samples are taken for serological reactions and the pathologist performs a full autopsy. If the reports of the serological examination and the pathologist are satisfactory, about a week after removal of the bones from the body these are denuded of remnants of muscle, ligaments and periosteum, and grafts of appropriate size are cut with a saw, specially constructed for this purpose and fitted with a water cooling device (fig. II.1 and II.2). The size of the grafts varies from 10 by 2 cm to 18 by 3 cm. Each graft is placed in a separate sterile jar (fig. II.3) and again stored in the deep-freeze. Samples are also taken for bacteriological investigation. If the culture is negative, the grafts become available for use.

The temperature of our deep-freeze during the period from 1953 till 1959 was —40° C; from 1959 till 1966 —55° C; from 1966 onward —90° C.

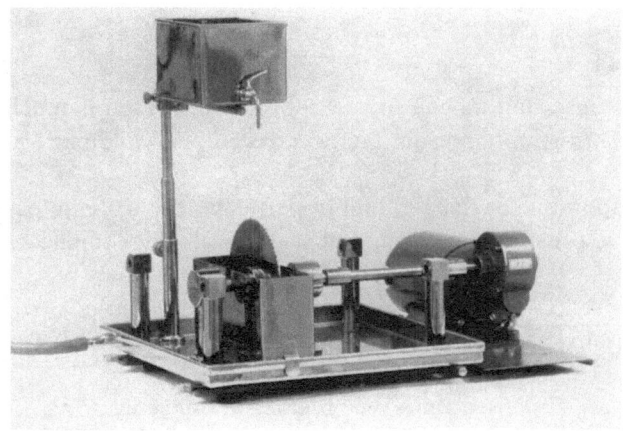

Figure II.1

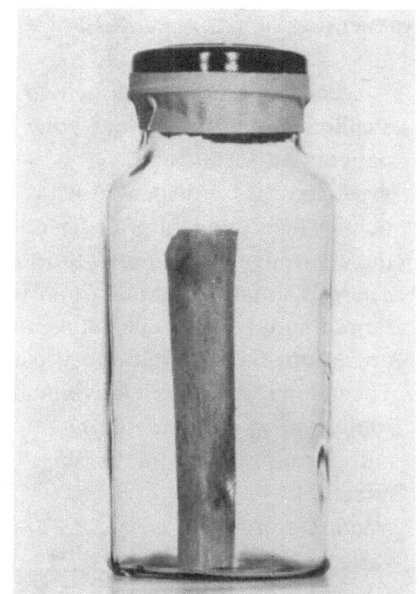

Figure II.3

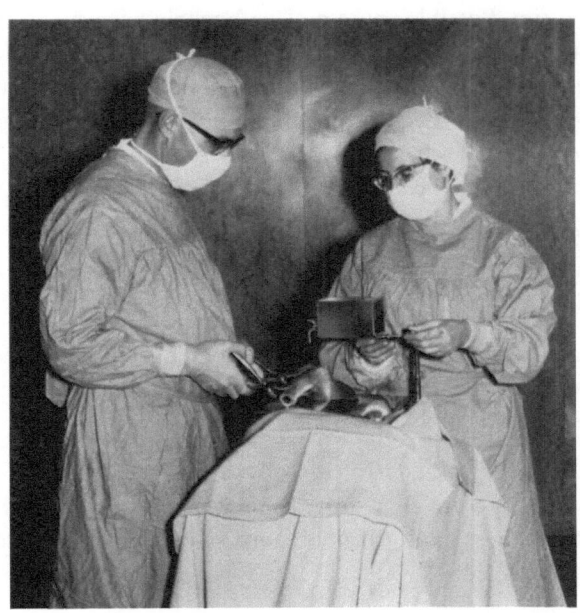

Figure II.2

ADVANTAGES OF THE BONE-BANK

1. A second operation is dispensed with, the operating time is shorter, and the operation is much smaller than if autogenous bone is used. This is an important factor, especially in children, e.g. patients with scoliosis.
2. A second scar is dispensed with; this is important for females and in particular for scoliotic patients where taking a graft from the iliac crest may leave a wound of scar, which will complicate the wearing of a Milwaukee brace.
3. There is ample material. Children, poliomyelitis patients, patients with multiple injuries often cannot supply sufficient autogenous material. The bone-bank can supply a large wide graft for operations such as a pseudarthrosis repair of the femur.
4. The complications of removing bone tissue are dispensed with. We observed in our series:
   complications at the donor site

autogenous grafts from the tibia	316
infection	4
fracture or fissure	7
varicose ulcer	1

DISADVANTAGES OF THE BONE-BANK

1. It is a laborious method, requiring much preliminary work and great care.
2. Danger of infection. Infection lies in wait at each orthopaedic operation; in bone transplantation the danger is particularly great as dead bone tissue, a good nutrient medium for bacteria, is left behind in the operation site. Possible sources of pathogenic bacteria at the site of operation are: non-sterility of the donor corpse, errors in removing or storing of the bones, and the violation of aseptic technique during surgery. Our patients, operated on with bone-bank grafts have been carefully observed, and records have been made of the post-operative course. *Undisturbed primary wound healing was observed in 271 cases, disturbances in wound healing in 4.*
   The details of the operations complicated by disturbed wound healing are as follows:

Male, 32 years old. 9–3–1956: operated on because of a pseudarthrosis of the tibia accompanying osteomyelitis. The cavity was cleared and filled with cancellous chips. After the operation recurrence of osteomyelitis occurred; the bone chips were removed later.

Male, 26 years old. Diagnosis: pseudarthrosis of the tibia, haemophilia; 29–5–1956: bone grafting operation, bone-bank chips applied; after the operation a large haematoma, wound dehiscention, secondary wound healing and healing of the pseudarthrosis.

Male, 30 years old. Diagnosis: pseudarthrosis of the femur, haemophilia; 9–11–1959: grafting with bone-bank graft; post-operatively a large haematoma occurred with rupture of the wound; on 14–12–1959 amputation was performed because of uncontrollable secondary bleeding; the patient recovered.

Male, 40 years old. Diagnosis: osteomyelitis of the femur; 16–10–1962 operated on: a large cavity in the femur was cleared and filled with cancellous bone-bank chips, post-operative course was initially satisfactory, but later on there was sinus formation with discharge of pus; the inserted bone chips had to be removed.

It appears from this summary that the disturbances in wound healing, 4 in 275 cases, can be reasonably attributed to the original lesion for which surgery was performed and were not caused by infection of the bone-bank tissue.
This data warrants the conclusion that the technique of sterile autopsy and storing the transplantation material at low temperatures and using meticulously aseptic techniques does not entail the risk of infection.

3. Danger of intolerance to the foreign tissue.

In transplantation of parenchymatous organs great problems arise because of the normal defence mechanisms. On the basis of clinical observation and experimental investigation we have suggested that the failure of heterogenous bone transplantation must be attributed, amongst other factors, to the defence mechanism of the host against the donor bone tissue. The question arises whether this factor plays a part in homogenous bone transplantation. In this respect too we have carefully observed our patients after our operation looking specifically for the possible occurrence of sensitivity reactions. After heterogenous bone transplantation (deep-freeze calf bone) we observed seromas and sinuses (Arch. Chir. Neerl. (1968) XII: 221); we have considered these phenomena to be manifestations of the defence mechanism. After homogenous bone transplantation we have not observed these phenomena.

We have, although realizing the theoretical drawbacks accompanying these proceedings, performed a second implantation of homogenous bone on several occasions at a varying time following the first operation. There were even a few patients who were given a homogenous graft three times.

225 patients received a homogenous graft once,
22 patients received a homogenous graft twice,
2 patients received a homogenous graft three times.

The patients who received a homogenous graft on three separate occasions were a girl with scoliosis, who was operated on in 3 stages and a boy with a recurring bone cyst.
We have observed no particular symptoms in our patients with the exception of the following three cases:

Patient no. 2, chapter IV, a boy with a solitary bone cyst, who was operated on three times. Each time cancellous homogenous bone was inserted. The boy suffered from bronchial asthma which first appeared at the age of 4, following the first operation.

Patient no. 5, chapter V, a man who sustained multiple injuries in a road accident. He was operated on many times and many drugs were administered, i.e. kemital, pethidine, macrodex, blood, ARS, AGS, TFT, penicillin, streptomycin, tetracycline, luminal atropine, soneryl; osteosynthesis with the aid of a homogenous graft was performed twice. During preparation for his 10th operation, after induction with kemital and pethidine, he went into a deep shock. Further investigation demonstrated that he was allergic to barbiturates and penicillin.

Patient no. 13, chapter V, a woman with a pseudarthrosis of the left humerus, had osteosynthesis performed with a homogenous graft. $1\frac{1}{2}$ years after this operation she was revaccinated against small-pox on the right arm; 3 weeks later the left arm became swollen and painful.

The question must be asked how far the implantation of homogenous tissue is liable to result in the development of these reactions. From what we know about the origin of these conditions they are all caused by many factors and the bone transplant may possibly have contributed to the occurrence of these reactions; but it would be incorrect to attribute these reactions solely to the bone transplant.

CONCLUSION

In our opinion, there is, from this point of view, no objection to the transplantation of homogenous bone. Although repeating this operation on the same patient must be advised against on theoretical grounds, we have observed no untoward results. However, it is recommended to use bone from a different donor in the case of a second or third implantation.

In the field of homogenous transplantations, the orthopaedic surgeon is in a more favourable position (shared with the ophthalmic surgeon performing transplantation of cornea) than his colleagues of other surgical disciplines with regard to transplantation of parenchymatous organs. This remarkable phenomenon may be attributed to various factors:

1. Bone transplantation is not a transplantation of living tissue, it is an implantation of dead tissue.
2. Bone tissue contains few antigenic substances; its antigenic properties are descreased by the deep-freeze procedure.
3. Cortical bone grafts are less antigenic than cancellous grafts. From the work of Burwell et al. it may be concluded that the antigenic activity originates from the substance of the cell nucleus. As cortical graft is poor in cell material and in addition the substance of the dead bone cell is only slowly released into the circulation of the host, there is little or no antigenic activity in cortical grafts.

Cancellous bone tissue is rich in cells, especially bone marrow cells which are situated between the trabeculae, hence cancellous bone does possess some antigenic activity. In this respect it is important to report that based on clinical observations we had already reached the conclusion that the application of fragments of cancellous bone from the bone-bank in fractures, pseudarthrosis, spondylodesis etc. did not have any favourable effect on osteogenesis; in these circumstances we advise against the use of cancellous bone from the bone-bank and we strongly caution against using this material if a second bone transplantation has to be performed.

CHAPTER III

STATISTICAL INFORMATION

During the period from 1–2–1953 until 1–2–1965, 958 operations using bone transplantation were performed by the authors and their collaborators.

An operation with bone transplantation is defined here as an operation in which one or more small or large fragments of bone tissue are inserted in the operative area. Strictly speaking it is not a transplantation, but an implantation; this procedure, however, is generally described as bone transplantation and therefore we have retained this expression.

These operations were performed in the Orthopaedic Department of the Wilhelmina Gasthuis (W.G.) in Amsterdam; in the Department of the 'Sociale Verzekeringsbank' of the Burgerziekenhuis, Amsterdam; in the Boerhaave Clinic, Amsterdam and in the general hospital Zonnestraal at Hilversum. Of these operations 519 were performed in the Wilhelmina Gasthuis, 320 in the Burgerziekenhuis, 85 in the Boerhaave Clinic and 34 in the general hospital Zonnestraal. The following types of bone transplant were used:

1. fresh autogenous transplant, taken from the tibia or the iliac crest in the shape of a graft or as cancellous chips;
2. deep-freeze autogenous transplant; in a few instances, for a two stage operation, the transplant was obtained at the first stage and stored at low temperatures in a sterile jar until use at the operation proper;
3. homogenous transplant; this was obtained by sterile postmortem dissection of suitable corpses, the transplants were stored at low temperatures in a sterile jar in the deep-freeze;
4. freeze dried homogenous transplant from the U.S. Navy Tissue Bank;
5. heterogenous transplant: calf bone preserved at low temperatures and supplied by the Bone Transplantation Service of the Netherlands Red Cross;
6. heterogenous transplant: modified calf bone, commercially available under the name of 'Kiel graft';
7. combinations were sometimes used.

Table III.1 shows the frequency with which the various types were used.

It is evident from table 1 that fresh autogenous and deep-freeze homogenous transplants were by far the most frequent type used; these two groups will be analyzed further; the other groups, owing to the small number of cases, are but of secondary importance in this investigation.

In studying the results of these operations, attention was paid to: wound healing, the frequency of infection, sinuses or sequestra, the transformation of the graft, and the consolidation.

It has been aimed to assess the result at least one year after the operation; in a number of cases

Table III.1. Various types of grafts used

fresh autogenous	647
homogenous	275
heterogenous	5
deep-freeze autogenous	9
autogenous and homogenous	10
freeze dried homogenous	5
autogenous and heterogenous	5
heterogenous kiel	2
total	958

where the result was quite obvious after a shorter time, a shorter period was accepted for practical purposes. E.g. after a fracture or pseudarthrosis the result was often obvious within the year.

A transplantation was rated as a success if a bony union had developed between the graft and the bone tissue of the patient and if the graft had been transformed into a living part of the host's skeletal system; if not the operation was rated as a failure.

A number of cases were met in which it was not possible to determine the end-result; this was caused by: some patients who did not turn up for the investigation, some patients were dead at this time, some data was of insufficient quality (especially X-ray photographs) to warrant a definite conclusion, or other uncertainties. It has been constantly aimed to limit this group to as small a number as possible. These cases are summarized under the heading 'unknown'.

In the present investigation the anatomical end-result of the operation is emphasized. The anatomical and clinical results usually correspond well; this is most clearly demonstrated in fractures and pseudarthroses. However, such a relationship does not occur in all cases, e.g. it is well-known that there are cases of spinal fusion with a perfect bony union but the patient has not improved and also the other way round, incomplete bony union with a contented patient. Table III.2 represents the over-all results.

Table III.2. Results of all operated cases

total	investigated	success	failure	succumbed	unknown
958	889 (93%)	766 (86%)	123	3	66 (7%)

Particular attention must be paid to three patients who died after the operation, the details of which follow below:

A woman aged 59. An arthrodesis of the right hip was performed on 25–7–1955 using a graft from the iliac crest. After-treatment in a plaster hip spica. 26–12–1955: sudden death occurred; post-mortem: pulmonary embolism.

A woman aged 48. At an accident on 10–9–1954 she sustained a fracture of the fore-arm. On 11–11–1955, because of pseudarthrosis of the radius and ulna, bone grafting was done using a graft from the patient's tibia. Sudden death occurred on 4–12–1955: post-mortem: pulmonary embolism.

A man aged 67. An arthrodesis of the left hip was performed on 11–2–1957 with a graft from the iliac crest. After-treatment in a plaster hip spica. On 5–3–1957 sudden death; post-mortem: pulmonary embolism.

Thus we have 3 patients who died as a result of a sudden massive pulmonary embolism; it must be noted that 2 of these had been treated in a plaster hip spica. After this experience all our patients eligible for treatment with anti-coagulants are given these drugs as a prophylactic measure. The post-operative mortality amounted to 3 cases, 0.3%, an exceptionally low percentage considering the large number of extensive operations. These results show that today it is possible to perform these extensive orthopaedic operations with a high degree of safety. The margin of safety will increase if one succeeds in preventing pulmonary embolism by the prophylactic administration of anti-coagulants. Apart from the right pre-operative conditioning of the patient, strict aseptic operative conditions, painstaking technique and proper aftertreatment, these very satisfactory results are without doubt largely due to modern anaesthesia and the dedication of our anaesthetists.

When discussing the risk attending an orthopaedic operation, one should also take into account the risk of post-operative complications, such as infection, which may invalidate the aim of the operation and even threaten the patient's life. This is all the more cogent, as orthopaedic operations are usually not life saving procedures. It is thus worthwhile to trace the post-operative complications in our series.

Table III.3. *Post-operative complications*

pulmonary embolism	6
necrosis of the skin	10
infection	13

Added to the 3 fatal cases of pulmonary embolism, the total number of cases of this amounts to 9, which is 1% of the number of operations. The occurrence of this dreaded complication in a frequency of 1% warrants prophylactic treatment with anti-coagulants.

The infections may be divided into 2 groups: 2 cases occurring in pre-operative 'clean' cases and 11 in cases that had already passed through an infected stage. In the latter the infection is most probably due to a flare up of the old infection; in the first group, however, the infection must be entirely due to the operation. Particular attention must be paid to the two cases in this group:

A man aged 39, lumbar spondylarthrosis. On 6–5–1953 a spinal fusion was performed using a graft from the patient's own tibia supplemented by calf bone chips from the bone-bank. Post-operative infection with a high temperature and suppuration of the wound occurred. Sequestrectomy had to be done subsequently.

A man aged 43, unstable back. On 17–11–1963 spinal fusion was performed with an autogenous tibial graft. Post-operative pain, fever, wound suppuration. On 3–5–1964, sequestrectomy.

It must be mentioned that a colleague had been present at the operation as a guest and that surgeon and guest had been engaged in a lively discussion. This experience has lead us to operate taciturnly and to stop demonstration operations. In table III.4 the complications arising at the site from which the graft was taken, have been enumerated below.

Table III.4. *Complications at the donor site*

infections	4	
fracture or fissure	7	= 2% of 316 tibial grafts
varicose ulcer	1	

The occurrence of tibial fractures after taking the graft has lead us to apply a plaster.

The 4 cases of infection, added to those 2 previously mentioned, give a total of 6 infections occurring in the 'clean' cases, that is 6 infections in 958 operations, 0.6%. The percentage of infection in these 'clean' operations thus amounted to 0.6%.

The results grouped accordingly to the type of transplant used, are shown in table III.5.

Table III.5. Results of the various types of transplant

	total	investigated	success	failure	succumbed	unknown
autogenous	647	599	519	80	2	46
homogenous	275	260	227	33	1	14
heterogenous	5	5	4	1	—	—
deep-freeze autogenous	9	8	5	3	—	1
autogenous and homogenous	10	4	3	1	—	6
freeze dried homogenous	5	5	5	—	—	—
autogenous and heterogenous	5	5	1	4	—	—
heterogenous kiel	2	2	1	1	—	—
total	958	888	765	123	3	67

It is generally accepted that autogenous transplantations give a better result than homogenous, and these again better than heterogenous. We are, with some reservations, of the same opinion, notwithstanding the fact that in our statistics homogenous transplantations show a slightly better outcome than the autogenous transplantations. This remarkable result is without a doubt due to the fact that experience has shown us which operations are most suitable for homogenous transplantation and at which operation an autogenous transplantation is to be preferred, in other words a selection has been made (see chapter II, page 94).

CHAPTER IV

FILLING-UP A CAVITY

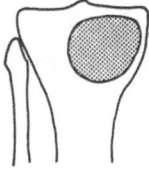

The following table presents statistical information regarding these operations in which a bone transplantation has been performed for filling-up a cavity.

Table IV.1. Filling-up a cavity

	total	investigated	success	failure	unknown	succumbed
autogenous	19	16	13	3	3	—
homogenous	35	28	23	5	7	—

Little value may be attached to this table unless it is split up into 'sterile' and 'infected' cavities. To the category sterile cavities belong solitary bone cysts, fibrous dysplasia, benign tumours and defects following trauma.

The category infected cavities arise as a consequence of infection. The following sub-division is made:

Sterile cavities:

	total	success	failure	unknown
autogenous	16	11	2	3
homogenous	31	21	3	7

Infected cavities:

	total	success	failure
autogenous	3	2	1
homogenous	4	2	2

The following examples illustrate these figures:

23

Diagnosis: solitary bone cyst of the right humerus.

Course:
13–10–1961:   operation: exposure of the shaft of the right humerus, opening up and curettage of the cyst, insertion of a homogenous graft into the cavity and fixation to cortical bone by means of one screw.
Post-operative course satisfactory, primary healing.
7–3–1963:   removal of screw.
5–12–1968:   reconstruction complete.

Examination:
5–12–1968:   normal form and function, no recurrence.

Radiographs:
3–1–1961:   figure IV.1a, cyst of the right humerus, near the epiphyseal cartilage.
28–8–1961:   figure IV.1b, condition before operation, cyst 'moved away' from epiphysis in the direction of the diaphysis.
13–10–1961:   figure IV.1c, condition after operation.
10–1–1963:   figure IV.1d, reconstruction of the shaft of the humerus.

Summary: Solitary bone cyst in a boy aged 8, treated by a homogenous bone graft; beautiful reconstruction of the shaft. With a long cortical graft.

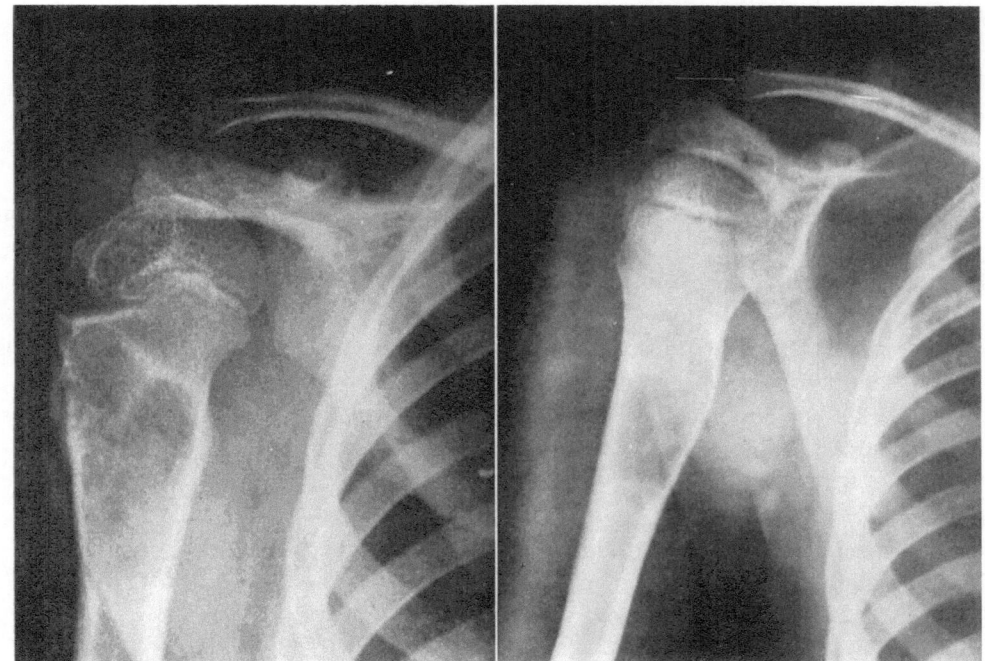

Figure IV.1a   Figure IV.1b

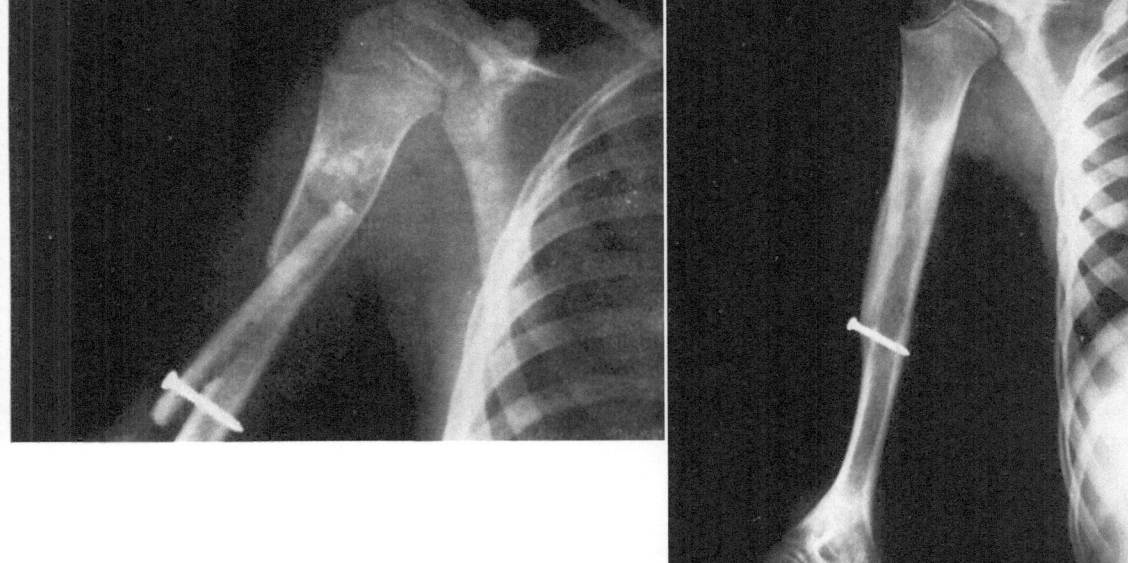

Figure IV.1c   Figure IV.1d

25

Diagnosis: solitary bone cyst of the right humerus.

Course:

15–11–1957: operation: curettage of the cyst, filling of the cavity with bits of cancellous homogenous bone.

16–1–1959: operated again because of recurrence, cavity filled up again with bits of cancellous homogenous bone.

25–3–1966: operated again because of recurrence, cavity now filled with bits of homogenous bone and a homogenous graft.

This boy suffered from bronchial asthma, which, according to his mother, started after the first operation.

Radiographs:

7–2–1966: figure IV.2a, cavity in the humeral shaft of the right arm.

8–6–1966: figure IV.2b, post-operative.

29–3–1967: figure IV.2c, very satisfactory result.

Summary: A solitary bone cyst in a boy aged 3, twice treated with cancellous grafting, and in whom the cyst recurred after each graft; the second recurrence was treated with a homogenous cortical graft, after which a very satisfactory result was obtained.

3 times a homogenous graft was performed. From this respect it is worth while mentioning that he suffers from bronchial asthma.

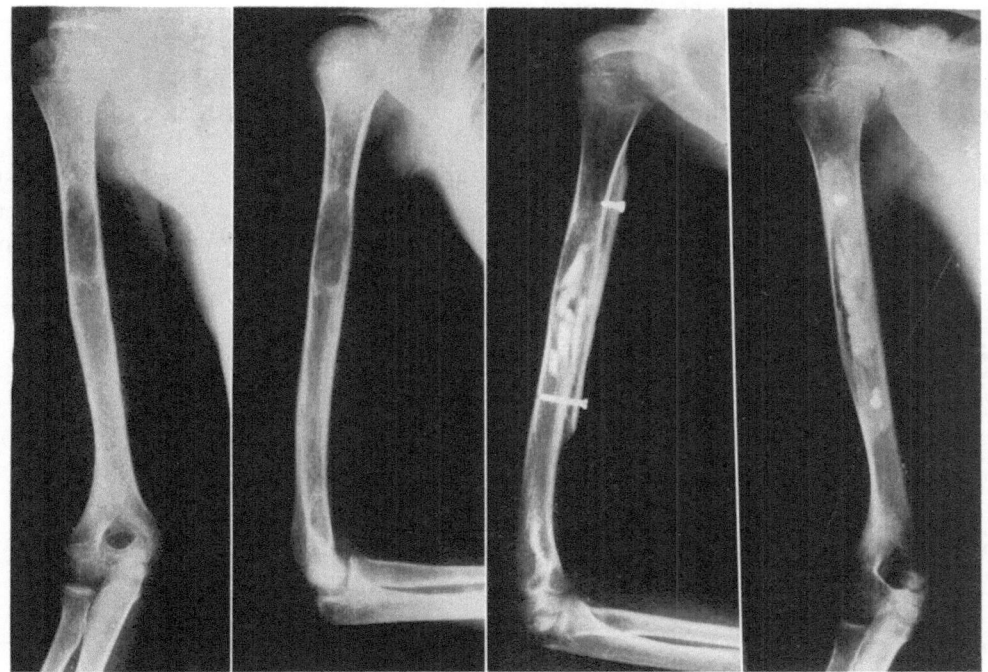

Figure IV.2a   Figure IV.2b

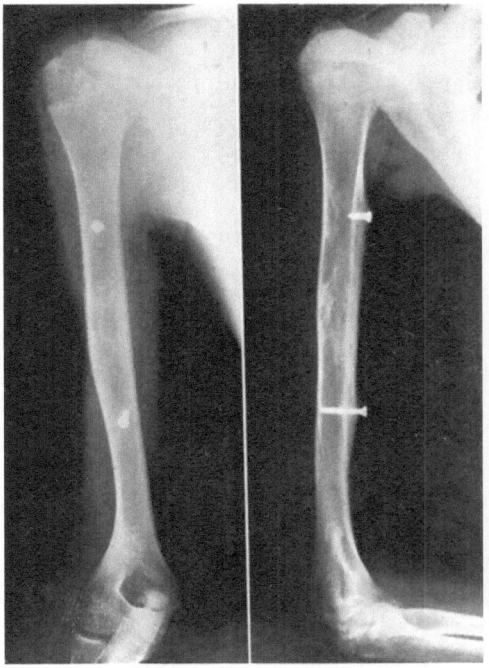

Figure IV.2c

27

Diagnosis: cyst of the right humerus.

Case history: disease started in 1953, cyst of the right humerus, operated on in 1953, the cyst was filled with autogenous bone chips from the iliac crest; in 1957 a fracture occurred through the cyst, after which he was referred to us because of the recurrence of the cyst with pseudarthrosis.

Course:
8–1–1958: operation: curettage of the cavity, freshening of the fracture, the cavity was filled with bits of cancellous homogenous bone, and a homogenous graft applied. Post-operative course satisfactory, primary healing.
10–4–1958: consolidation, no cyst.

Examination:
22–1–1969: no recurrence.

Radiographs:
11–3–1954: figure IV.3a, cyst of the right humerus.
17–12–1957: figure IV.3b, cyst of the right humerus and pseudarthrosis.
8–4–1958: figure IV.3c, healed after bone grafting.
22–1–1969: figure IV.3d, last X-ray.

Summary: Cyst of right humerus, recurrence with pseudarthrosis in a boy aged 10, healed after homogenous bone grafting.

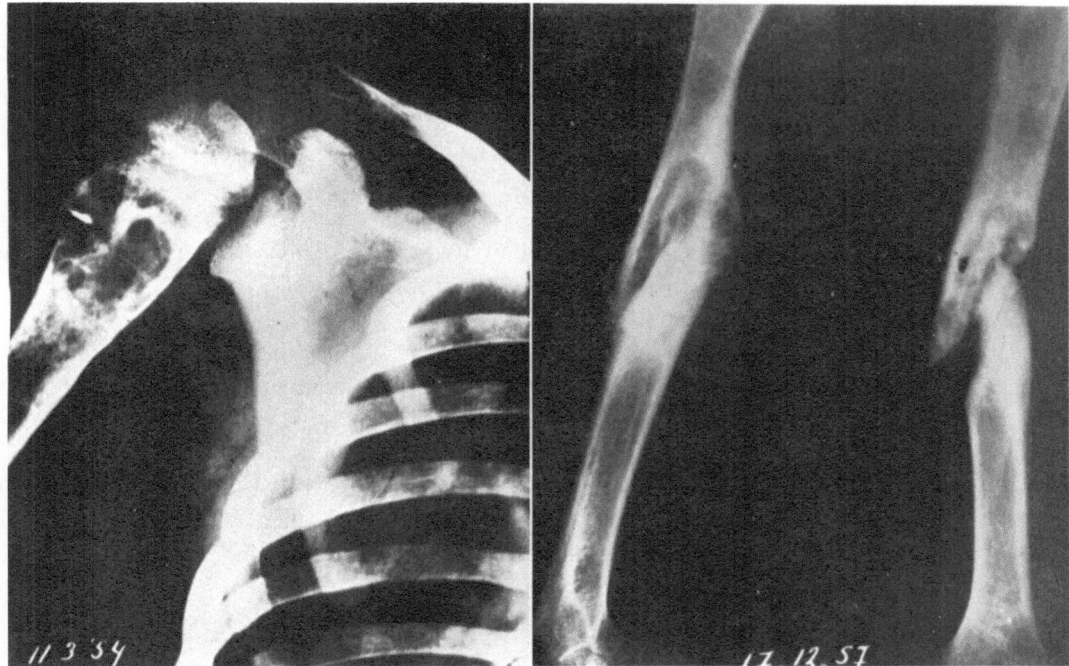

Figure IV.3a   Figure IV.3b

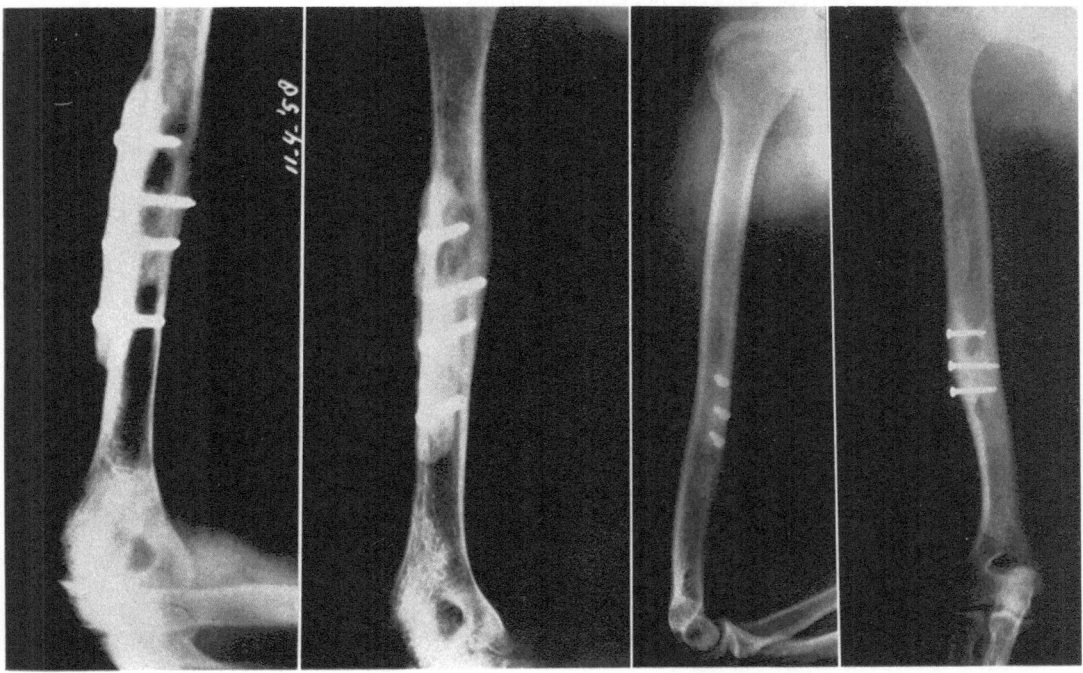

Figure IV.3c   Figure IV.3d

29

Diagnosis: solitary bone cyst of left humerus.

Case history:

10–1–1945:   fracture, treated with skin traction.

2–11–1951:   operation elsewhere, curettage of the cavity in the proximal part of the left humerus, and filling-up with autogenous bone tissue from iliac crest.

6–7–1959:   refracture through the cyst.

31–8–1959:   admission to the Orthopaedic Department of Wilhelmina Gasthuis because of a large solitary bone cyst of the left humerus with accompanying fracture.

Course:

7–9–1959:   operation: opening up and curettage of the cyst, which was 8 cm long; a homogenous graft was jammed into the cyst, and the remaining cavity filled with chips of cancellous homogenous bone. After-treatment with balanced skin traction.
Post-operative course satisfactory, primary healing.

Radiographs:

15–7–1959:   figure IV.4a, cyst with fracture, left humerus.

11–1–1960:   figure IV.4b, 4 months after operation, graft visible.

27–2–1964:   figure IV.4c, no cyst visible, graft assimilated.

Summary: Solitary bone cyst of the left humerus in a female aged 26, with recurrence and fracture, very satisfactory result after treatment with homogenous graft.

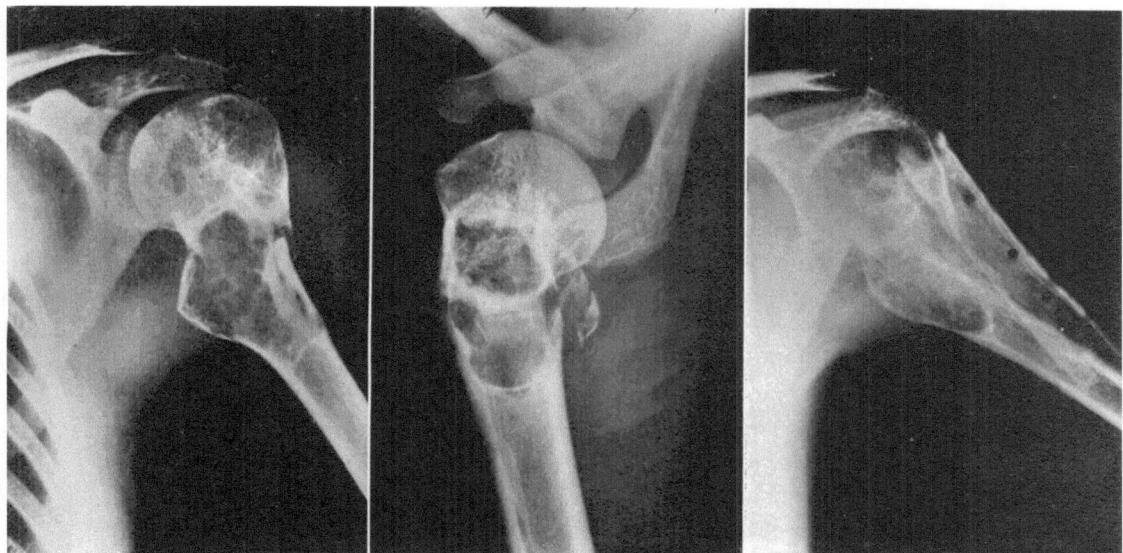

Figure IV.4a   Figure IV.4b

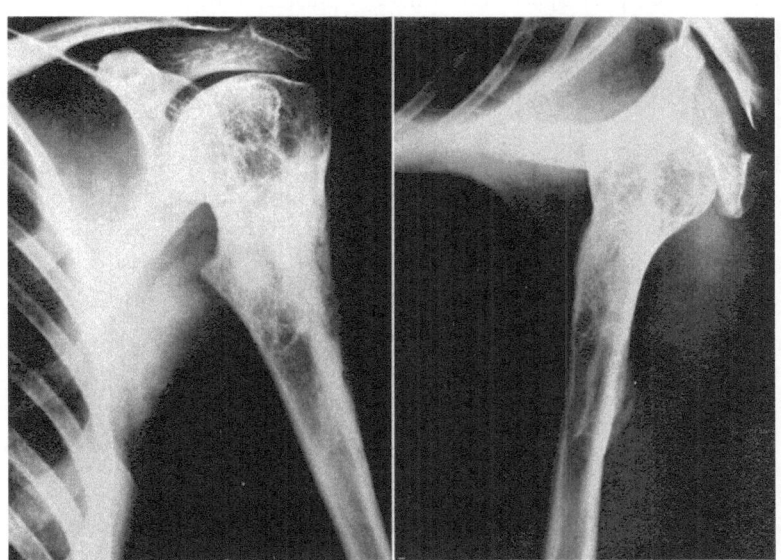

Figure IV.4c

Diagnosis: benign tumour of left femur.

Course:

3-12-1960: operation to expose the lateral side of the left femur, showing the presence of a spontaneous fracture. A cavity 3 cm long was filled with reddish brown elastic tissue. This cavity was curetted, and a homogenous graft inserted, one end of which was pointed and driven home proximally into the spongy bone, with the graft laid in the cavity and fixed distally to the cortical bone with one screw. After-treatment was in a hip spica.

Pathological examination showed the tumour to be a variant of local osteitis fibrosa and giant cell tumour, benign.

Post-operative course was satisfactory with primary healing.

15-3-1963: operation: removal of screw, no cavity perceptible.

Examination:

9-1-1968: good form and function of extremity, no recurrence of tumour.

Radiographs:

30-12-1960: figure IV.5a, post-operatively through plaster, showing a defect in the femur, 5 cm long, with the graft in situ and the overlying defect.

17-5-1961: figure IV.5b, graft visible.

1-2-1967: figure IV.5c, frontal, and figure IV.5d, med. lat., both good form.

Summary: Benign bone tumour in a boy aged 4, treated with a homogenous graft, no recurrence of tumour, very satisfactory reconstruction of the femoral shaft.

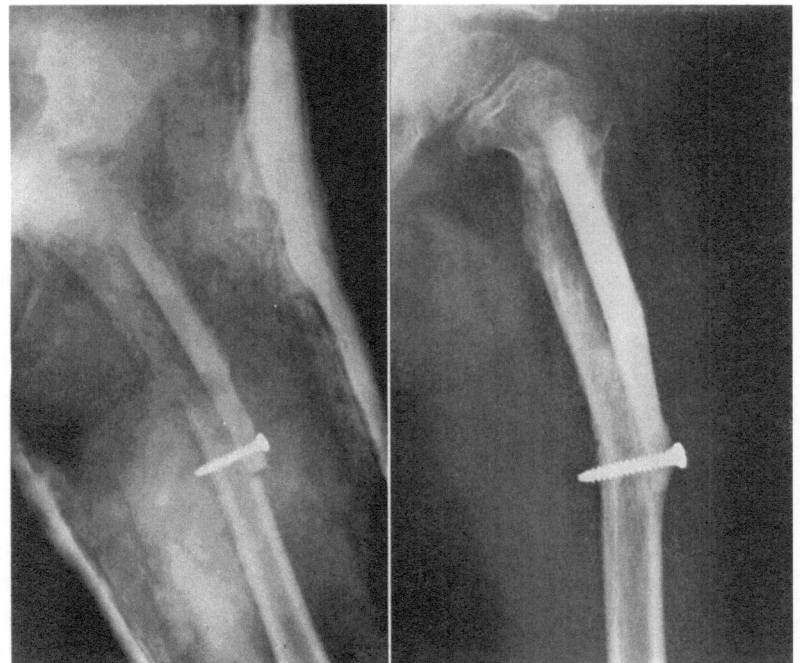

Figure IV.5a   Figure IV.5b

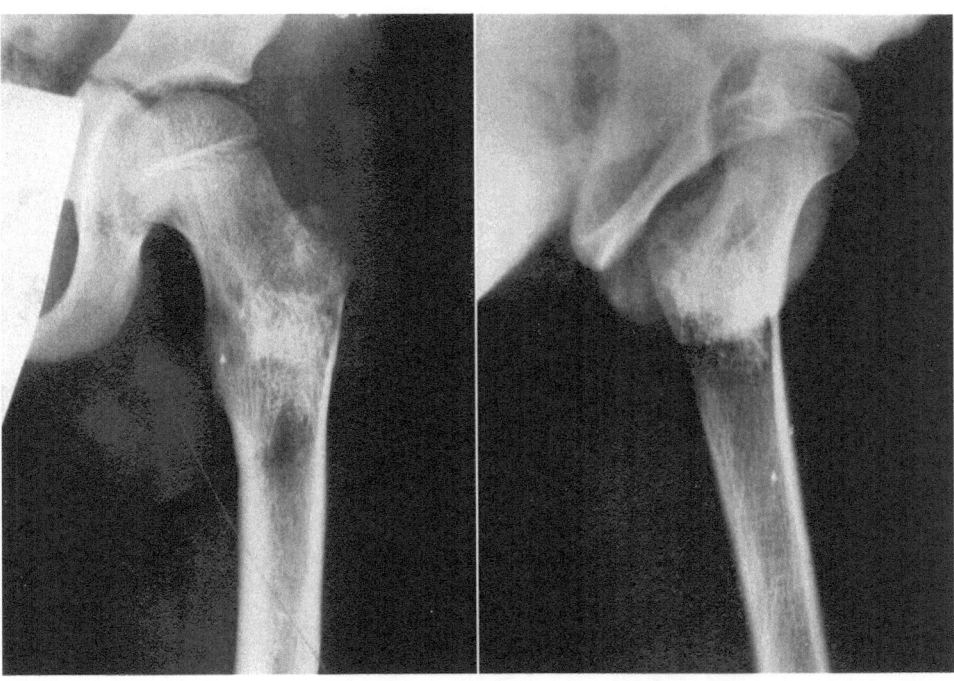

Figure IV.5c   Figure IV.5d

33

Diagnosis: fibrous dysplasia in right femur with spontaneous fracture.

Course:
14–6–1963:   operation: diagnostic biopsy, which on pathological examination showed the tumour to be fibrous dysplasia.
11–7–1963:   operation: emptying of the cavity, insertion of a homogenous graft, the remainder of the cavity was filled with pieces of autogenous bone from the iliac crest.
Post-operative course satisfactory, primary healing.

Radiographs:
18–5–1963:   figure IV.6a, large cavity in the proximal part of right femur.
11–7–1963:   figure IV.6b, post-operative: graft visible.
6–6–1966:   figure IV.6c, satisfactory assimilation of the graft.

Summary: Man, 38 years old with a large cavity in the right femur, caused by *fibrous dysplasia*, treated with a combination of a homogenous graft and autogenous cancellous bone with a very satisfactory result. The period of observation was short, since he did not turn up for further examination.

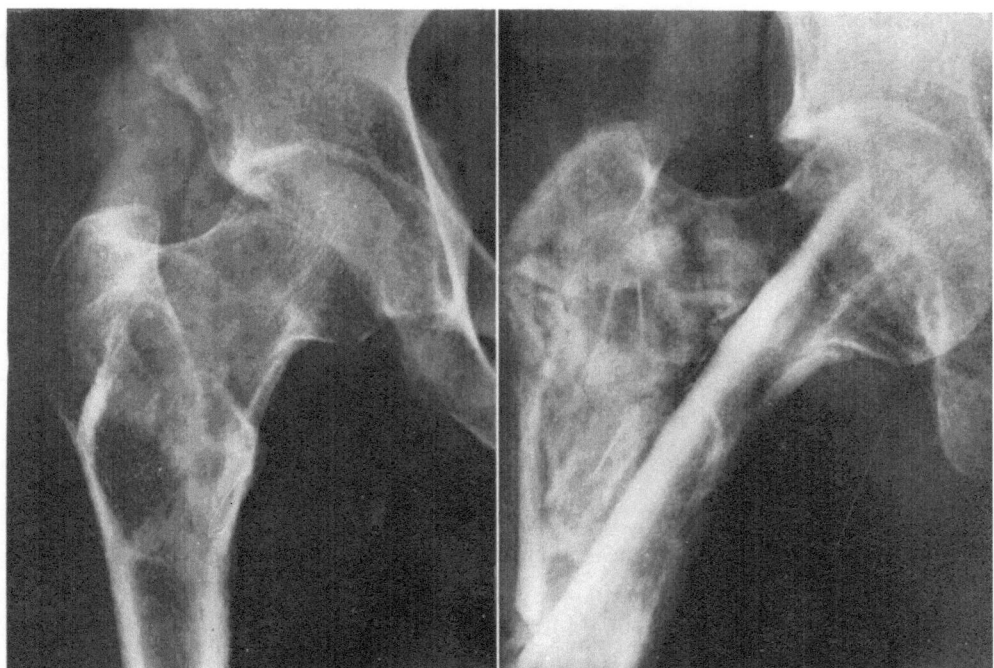

Figure IV.6a   Figure IV.6b1

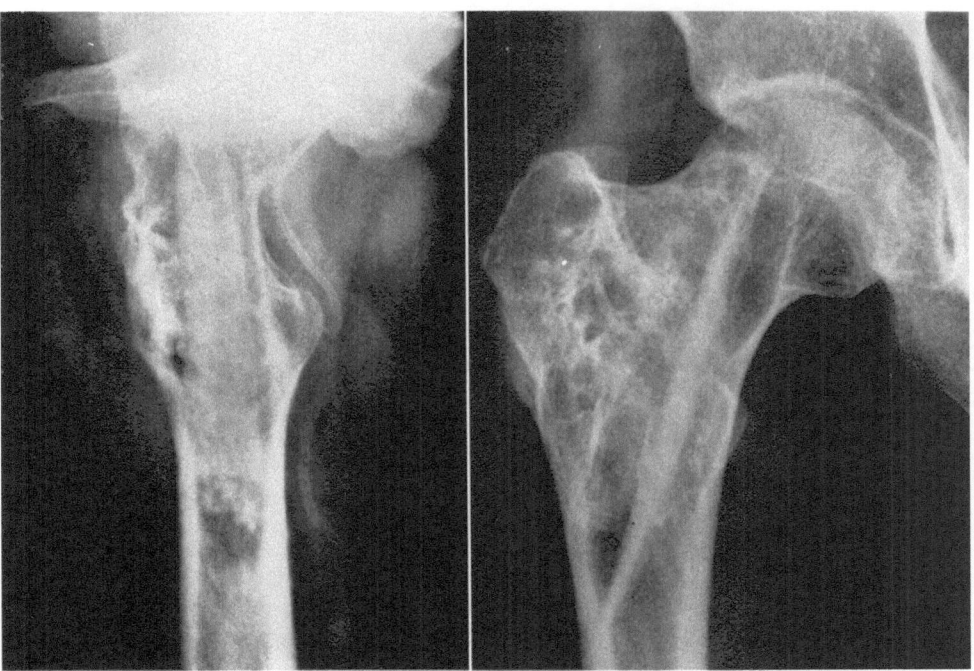

Figure IV.6b2   Figure IV.6c

35

Diagnosis: giant cell tumour of the right femur.

Course:
12–4–1960:   operation: opening up of the cavity which contained yellowish-red soft elastic tissue. After curettage the cavity was filled with small fragments of cancellous homogenous bone.
Post-operative course satisfactory, primary healing.
Pathological examination: a giant cell tumour.

Examination:
10–10–1968:   good condition.

Radiographs:
19–3–1960:   figure IV.7a, cavity in the medial femoral condyle, $5 \times 7 \times 5$ cm.
12–4–1960:   figure IV.7b, post-operative, cavity filled with transplanted bone.
10–10–1968:   figure IV.7c, good assimilation of transplanted bone, no recurrence of tumour.

Summary: *Giant cell tumour* in a male aged 35, treated with fragments of cancellous homogenous bone; very satisfactory result.

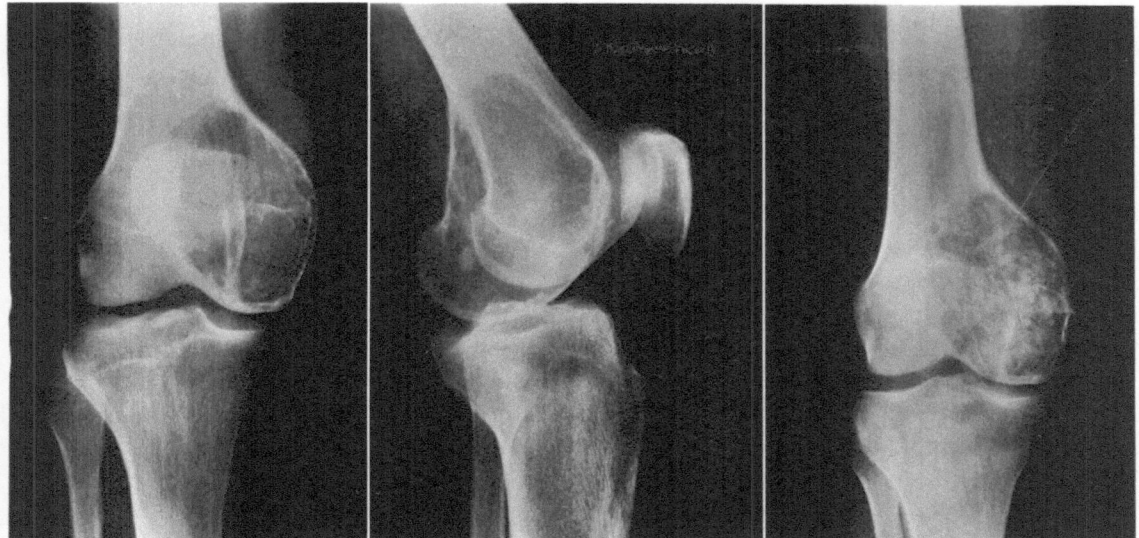

Figure IV.7a

Figure IV.7b1

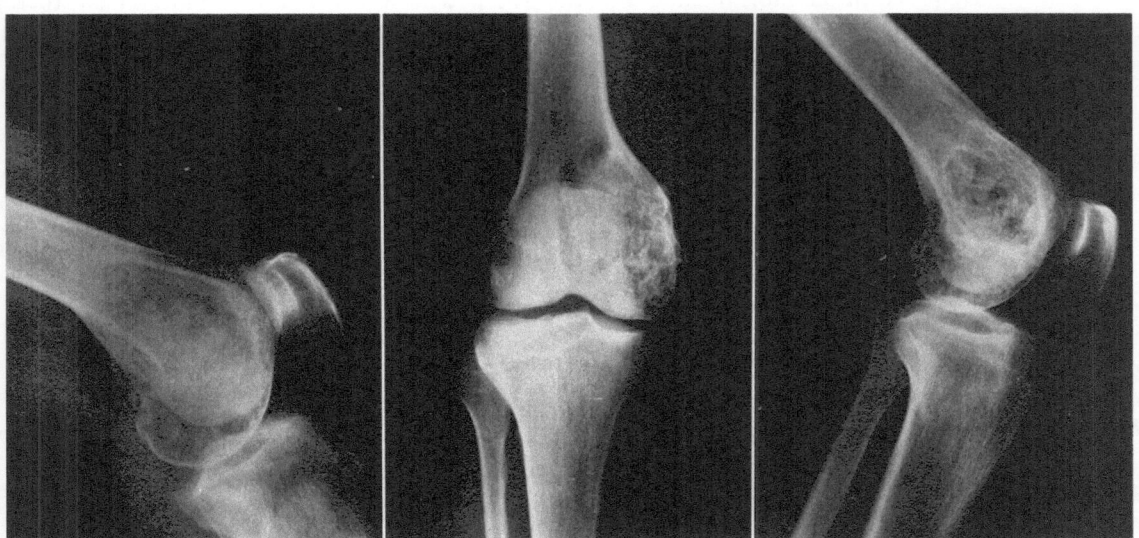

Figure IV.7b2

Figure IV.7c

PATIENT IV.8, MALE, BORN 8–5–1922

Diagnosis: from September 1960 osteomyelitis of the distal right femur, the cause of which was not obvious.

Course:

Sept./Oct. 1960:   observation.

Dec. 1960/Jan. 1961:   after exploration, osteomyelitis was diagnosed.

June/July 1961:   operative treatment.

Aug./Dec. 1961:   hospitalization because of discharge from the operation wound.

Oct. 1962/Febr. 1963:   in Orth. Dept. W.G.

16–10–1962:   curettage of the cavity, which was filled with homogenous bone chips, closure of the wound. Continuous 'drip and suck' drainage with penicillin, parenteral penicillin and streptomycin.

28–12–1962:   excision of the sinus track. Curettage of the cavity, which was the size of a mandarin. Closure of the wound. Continuous drip and suck drainage.

31–1–1963:   discharged home; sinus still present with discharge of pus. Pathological examination: non-specific, subacute inflammation.

21–4–1964:   admission; sinus quiescent. Haemoglobin 100%, ESR 15 mm/1st hour. Urine normal. Muscle-plasty operation considered.

15–12–1966:   Treatment in hyperbaric chamber (Boerema) 100 hours, without improvement.

27–6–1969:   After prolonged walking there was still some discharge from the sinus. Dressings renewed in the morning and at night. The patient was lean, although never fat, there is evidence of weight loss. However, he leads a normal life, aiding his wife in a shop. He has a full disability allowance, the factory pays for his pension, and he also gets a holiday allowance. His weight was 128 kg.

His heart was not enlarged, there was no oedema. Pulmonary function normal. Spleen not enlarged. Pulse rate 75, equal, no hypertension. The leg was not swollen. Along the posterior edge of the tensor muscles a pencil thick induration was present. The scar was retracted by the pressure of a sinus. There was a discharge present on the dressing the size of half-a-crown. Function of the knee: complete extension, flexion up to 65°.

Bad result because the soft tissues are not sound, especially the skin and so the cavity could not be closed. Conclusion: retention – and infection –.

Light photographs: figure IV.8a, result.

Radiographs: 8–9–1966: figure IV.8b, result.

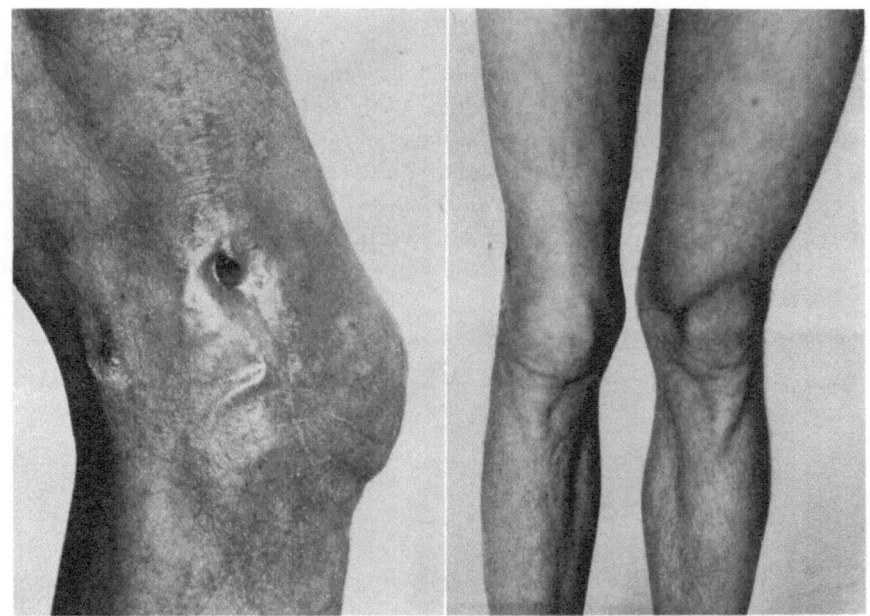

Figure IV.8a

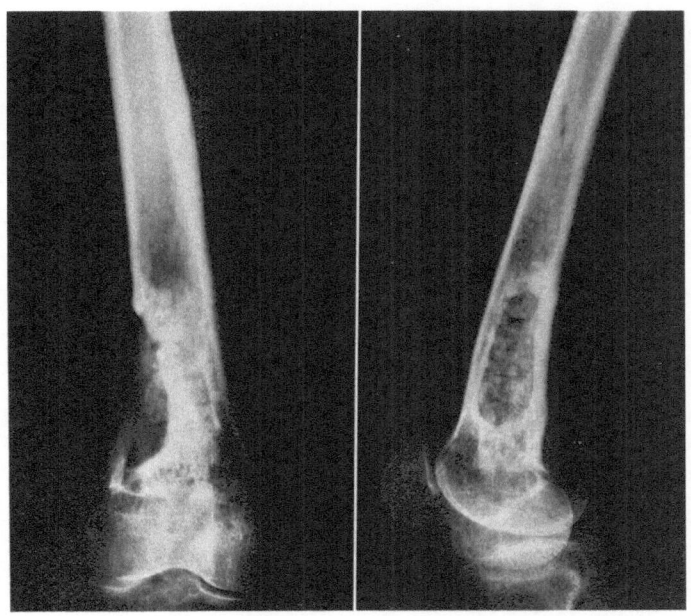

Figure IV.8b

CONCLUSION

Filling-up a cavity is a good indication for the use of homogenous bone. However, a clear distinction must be made between 'sterile' and 'infected' cavities. With 'sterile' cavities the results are excellent, with 'infected' cavities there are naturally a large number of failures. We are therefore of the opinion that homogenous bone must not be used in infected cavities.

The solitary bone cysts present a separate problem because of their tendency to recur. From clinical experience, we think that in these cases a homogenous cortical graft is more satisfactory than cancellous bone. The good results obtained from treating fibrous dysplasia and the giant cell tumour are very interesting.

CHAPTER V

GRAFT ALONGSIDE RECIPIENT BONE

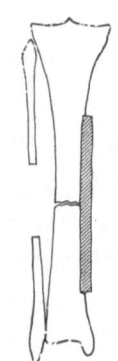

Scheme V.1

In this group are operations on the long bones, such as bone grafting in recent fractures, in pseudarthroses, and operations on joints such as intra- and para-articular arthrodeses, particularly spinal fusions.

Examples of recent fractures: patient V.1 up to and including V.7.
Examples of pseudarthrosis: patient V.8 up to and including V.13.
Examples of intra- and para-articular arthrodesis: patient V.14 up to and including V.18.
Examples of spinal fusion: patient V.19 up to and including V.21.

Table V.1. Statistics

autogenous	total	investigated	success	failure	unknown	succumbed
arthrodesis	259	242	206	36	16	1
spinal fusion	98	85	72	13	13	—
recent fracture	15	14	13	1	—	—
pseudarthrosis	193	185	163	22	7	1
homogenous	total	investigated	success	failure	unknown	succumbed
arthrodesis	16	14	12	2	1	1
spinal fusion	62	60	50	10	2	—
recent fracture	75	73	70	3	2	—
pseudarthrosis	71	70	61	9	1	—
pseudarthroses	total	investigated	success	failure	unknown	succumbed
autogenous	193	185	163 (88%)	22	7	1
homogenous	71	70	61 (87%)	9	1	—

CONCLUSION

This group should be considered suitable for the use of homogenous grafts.

RECENT FRACTURES

73 cases of recent fractures were treated by operative reduction and fixation with a homogenous cortical graft, 70 of the 73 operations were successful with bony consolidation of the fracture, 3 were registered as failures.

Analysis of the failures

Male, aged 32, the graft did not proceed to bony union with the recipient bone of the host, the fracture showed an extremely slow healing.

Boy, aged 9, patient V.4, the graft fractured, probably during transport to another hospital 4 weeks after the operation. The fracture healed with angulation. This observation is instructive in that a bank-bone graft must be protected against too great a stress.

Male, aged 34, patient V.5, this third case is a real failure, pseudarthrosis followed because of unstable osteosynthesis on account of a poor operative technique.

It should not remain unrecorded that a number of patients with a fracture, treated by osteosynthesis with a homogenous graft, *sustained a refracture*, although we are convinced there was complete healing of the original fracture. This phenomenon occurred in 4 out of the 73 patients. Two of these patients were suffering from osteogenesis imperfecta, one patient was transported prematurely to another hospital, 4 weeks after the operation (patient V.4), and in one patient it was probably a spontanous fracture (patient V.6).

PSEUDARTHROSIS

71 cases of pseudarthrosis were treated with a homogenous graft; 61 of the 71 operations were successful, that is 87%, 9 were rated as failure, and the outcome of one was unknown.

Table V.2. Pseudarthrosis

number	investigated	success	failure	unknown	succumbed
71	70	61	9	1	0

Analysis of the failures

Male, aged 23: fore-arm, ulna healed, radius pseudarthrosis.

Male, aged 41: humerus, fracture of the graft 6 months after operation.

Male, aged 29: humerus, fracture of the graft 6 months after operation.

Male, aged 43: radius, fracture of the graft 6 months after operation.

Male, aged 16: congenital pseudarthrosis of the tibia, this persisted.

Male, aged 43: humerus, fracture of the graft 5 months after operation.

Male, aged 28: femur, fracture of the graft 5 months after operation.

Male, aged 40: femur, fracture of the graft 16 months after operation.

Male, aged 44: femur, persistance of pseudarthrosis.

It appears from these observations that the fixation of the homogenous graft has been overrated in some cases because of the very slow initiation of biological activity by the homogenous graft.

Insufficient fixation combined with this slow initiation of biological activity are the cause of slow healing, refracture and pseudarthrosis. Because of this there must be a meticulous fixation technique with closely fitting planes of contact. After-treatment should be prolonged permitting only minimal stress. It is worth while to consider performing osteosynthesis with a homogenous graft using the A.O. compression principle.

In the group of pseudarthroses there was one, in which the pseudarthrosis proceeded to bony consolidation, with a subsequent spontaneous fracture.

This observation of spontaneous fractures (2 in 144 cases) *poses the question whether the quality of the callus in the vicinity of a homogenous graft might not be of inferior quality in some instances.*

ARTHRODESIS

The aim of arthrodesis is to create a bony ankylosis of a joint in a favourable position. The surgeon will have to adapt his technique according to circumstances. A joint damaged by inflammation has a natural tendency to proceed to fibrous ankylosis; a bone graft applied in the right way may provide preliminary fixation attended by biological activity which leads to bony ankylosis. According to circumstances, the graft may be placed inside the joint, alongside the joint or outside the joint (intra-, para- or extra-articular). With a joint damaged by osteoarthritis or with a sound joint that must be stabilized e.g. because of paralysis, it is more difficult to obtain bony ankylosis, a graft by itself will not be sufficient, and in these cases, the joint cartilage etc. must be removed back to cancellous bone to provide a physiological basis for vascularization. With arthrodesis the bone graft has a double function: firstly fixation, secondly to stimulate biological activity in the right way. If fixation by means of the graft only is insufficient then mechanical fixation will be necessary as well (patient no. 18, chapter V).

In general, '*biological reaction*' is best provided by an autogenous graft; the greater number of arthrodeses performed by us were consequently done with an autogenous bone graft.

Table V.3. Regarding arthrodesis

	total	investigated	success	failure	unknown	succumbed
autogenous	259	242	206	36	16	1
homogenous	16	14	12	2	1	1

All wrist-, knee-, ankle- and subtalar arthrodeses, with a few exceptions, have been performed using an autogenous graft.

We have used the homogenous graft successfully as an intra- or para-articular graft in cases of quiescent tuberculous arthritis and also to stabilize joints following poliomyelitis. The homogenous graft is not suitable for bridging a defect, consequently it is not suitable for extra-articular arthrodesis, *at least not in adults.*

SPINAL FUSION

This is a special type of arthrodesis. Here one must take into account the nature of the disease and the age of the patient.

There is a great difference between a vertebral column affected by tuberculous spondylitis, a vertebral column in an adult with degenerative disease and a vertebral column in a child with scoliosis.

The aim of spinal fusion in tuberculous spondylitis is not only to provide fixation, but above all to initiate biological reconstructive activity around the graft and the vertebral disease. For this purpose autogenous grafts must be used exclusively.

Creating a bony ankylosis of the vertebral column in an adult because of a degenerative disease is fraught with difficulties; it requires meticulous technique and only autogenous bone can awaken the high biological reactions under these circumstances.

It is entirely a different matter to bring about a spinal fusion in a child with idiopathic scoliosis. This type of scoliosis is a problem in itself. It is beyond the scope of this publication to enter into the many aspects of this problem, its aetiology, prognosis, conservative treatment, indications for operation, technique, after-treatment, and results. We shall confine ourselves to a description of our treatment, stating our results. A child with scoliosis, in which operative treatment is indicated, is admitted to hospital, put to bed with head and leg traction, whilst a Milwaukee brace is made. When the brace is ready and the child used to wearing it, the operation is performed.

Immediately before the operation the brace is removed. The operation is performed in the following manner: anaesthesia, prone position, longitudinal incision in the midline at the level of the primary curve of the scoliosis, subperiosteal exposure of the dorsal spinous processes, laminae, the articular processes and the transverse processes of the selected vertebrae. In general, the vertebrae of the primary curve with one above and one below are dealt with; in cases of paralytic scoliosis usually more vertebrae are involved. The intervertebral facet joints are opened up, curettage of these joints performed and a bone plug inserted, the dorsal spinous processes, the laminae, the transverse processes are stripped of the outer layer of cortical bone; these bone chips are arranged in a tile-like fashion about the intervertebral facet joints and *on either side* of the vertebral column small grafts of homogenous bone are placed in the angle between the dorsal spinous processes and the laminae. Post-operatively the patient is nursed alternatively prone, supine, on the right and on the left side. Two to three days after the operation the Milwaukee brace is put on again, and during the following days by lengthening the brace the scoliosis is corrected. Bed rest in the horizontal posture follows for 6 months, followed by gradual mobilization in a rehabilitation centre. Twelve months later the child is allowed back to school, but keeps the brace for a further 6–12 months. This operation is in fact a spinal fusion at 3 levels: firstly the interarticular arthrodesis of the small facet joints, secondly the layer of autogenous bone chips, and thirdly the homogenous grafts.

Judging the result of a spinal fusion is a separate problem. The criteria used are: the findings of the clinical and X-ray investigations, the amount of correction, the maintenance of the correction, and the development of a pseudarthrosis. There is by no means unanimity in the literature as regards the frequency of pseudarthrosis developing after a spinal fusion; it also depends on the diligence with which it is looked for.

In judging the result of our operations we relied on the clinical examination, the standard X-ray photographs and X-ray photographs with lateral bending. We attach great importance to good oblique radiographs of the operated area. We rated a spinal fusion as a success if according to this information the vertebral column showed a bony ankylosis; if mobility or a pseudarthrosis could be demonstrated we rated the operation as a failure.

From a total of 62 patients 60 were examined, 50 of these were registered as a success and 10 as failures; it must be pointed out that over the years we have gradually improved on our technique. This is noticeable in the results of the operations.

We think, on the basis of the cases demonstrated, that we have shown that homogenous grafts are a valuable aid in the treatment of scoliosis in children.

We intend to report in detail on these problems in a few years time when these patients will be adults.

CONCLUSION

This group, graft alongside bone, can be a relatively good indication for the use of a homogenous bone graft. In recent fractures of the long bones the possibility of applying a homogenous graft must be kept in mind, the results are good, in some conditions this type of graft is extremely useful.

The same applies to pseudarthroses, in some cases of pseudarthrosis the homogenous graft is an indispensable aid. In performing arthrodeses the autogenous graft is to be preferred; in selected cases such as quiescent arthritis the homogenous graft may be successfully used, the homogenous graft is not suitable for extra-articular arthrodesis.

The use of homogenous graft in spinal fusion in adults must be strongly advised against. In treating scoliosis in children the homogenous graft is extremely valuable.

We would now like to demonstrate the different indications.

PATIENT V.1, MALE, BORN 14–7–1937

Diagnosis: fracture of the right femoral shaft.

Course:
28–3–1963:   accident, admission to the Orth. Dept. W. G, fracture of the right femoral shaft.
9–4–1963:   operation: osteosynthesis using a homogenous graft. Post-operative course satisfactory, primary healing.
12–9–1963:   consolidation.

Examination:
24–10–1967:   excellent form and function of the right thigh.

Radiographs:
1–4–1963:   figure V.1a, long spiral fracture of the right femural shaft.
9–4–1963:   figure V.1b, post-operative.
14–9–1963:   figure V.1c, consolidation.
24–10–1967:   figure V.1d, bony consolidation between graft and femur.

Summary: Fracture of the shaft of the right femur in a male aged 25, osteosynthesis with the aid
of a bone-bank graft, excellent result.

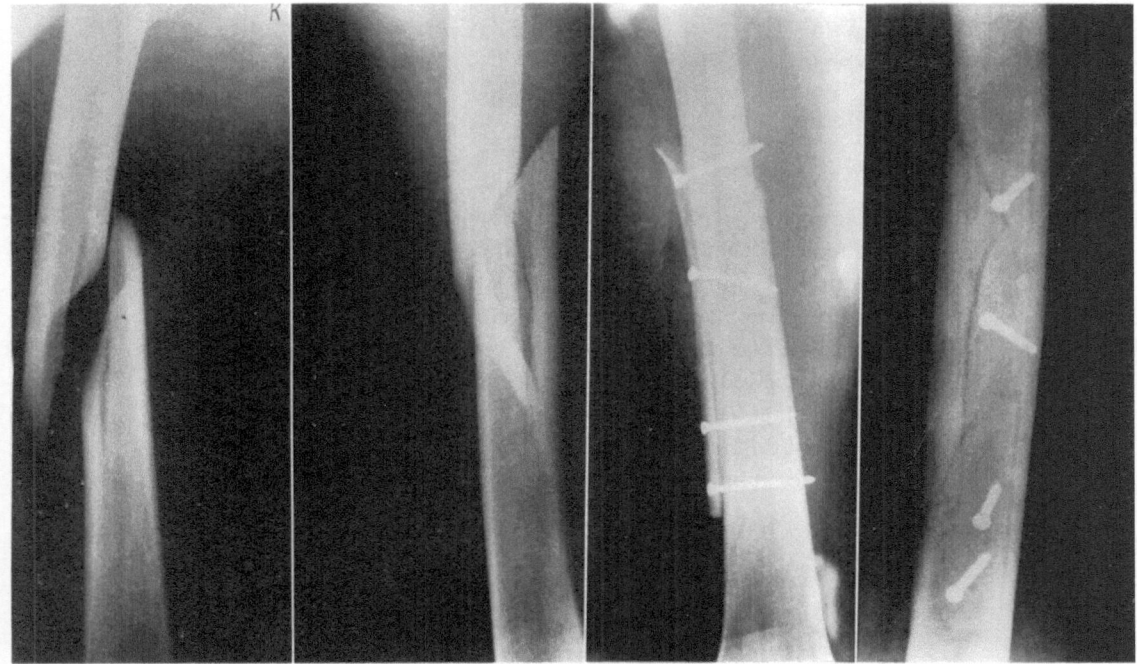

Figure V.1a   Figure V.1b

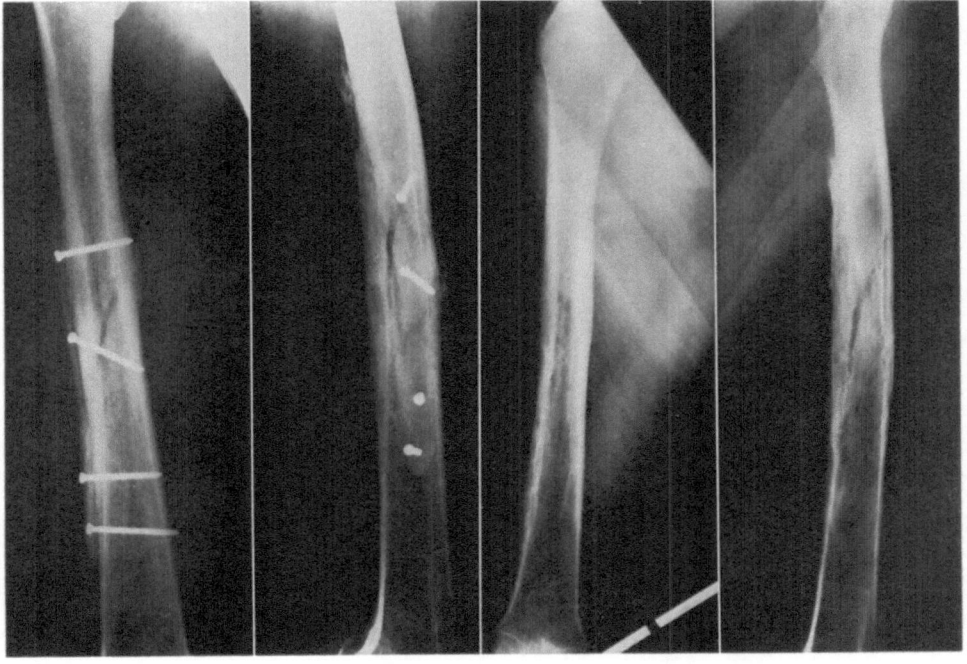

Figure V.1c   Figure V.1d

Diagnosis: multiple injuries.

Course:

16–12–1959:   motor-cycle accident, admitted to Orth. Dept. W.G., concussion, compound fracture of the left femoral shaft, subcapital fracture of the neck of the left femur, non-penetrating abdominal injury.

30–12–1959:   rupture of the spleen, laparotomy, splenectomy.

1–2–1960:   osteosynthesis of the neck of the femur with a Smith-Petersen nail, osteosynthesis of the fracture of the left femoral shaft with the aid of a homogenous graft. Post-operative course satisfactory, primary healing.

5–8–1960:   consolidation of the fractures, mobilized with non-weight bearing.

7–3–1961:   operation: removal of 2 screws and biopsy taken from graft.

Examination:

12–5–1966:   good form and function of left thigh.

Radiographs:

28–12–1959:   figure V.2a, fracture of left femoral shaft, fracture of neck of left femur.

20–2–1960:   figure V.2b, post-operative.

4–8–1960:   figure V.2c, consolidation.

12–5–1966:   figure V.2d, latest X-ray.

Continuation on page 50

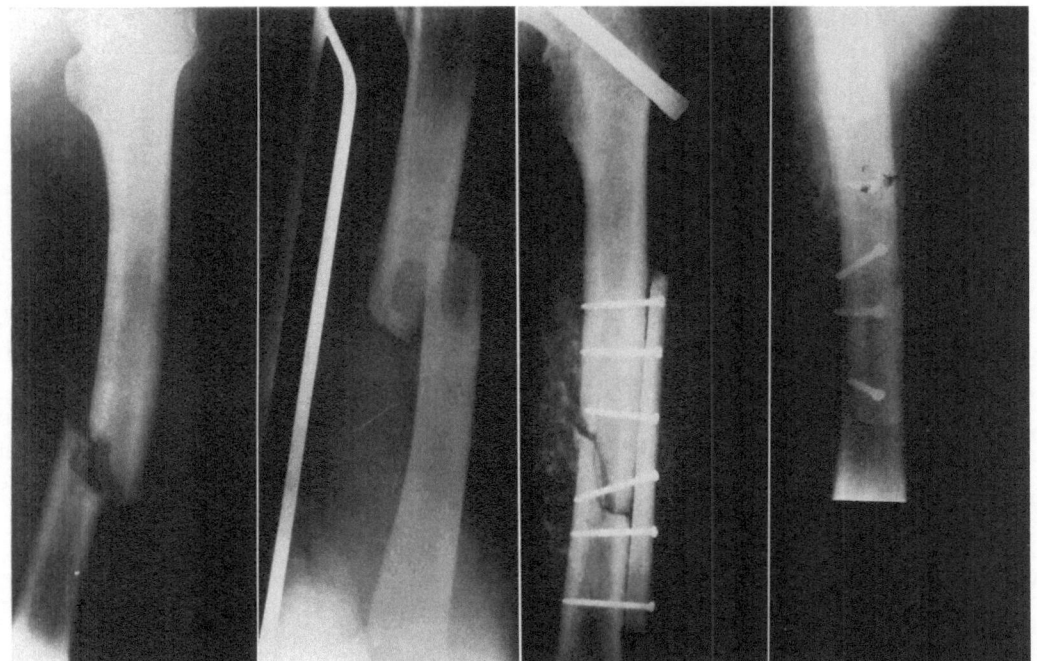

Figure V.2a   Figure V.2b

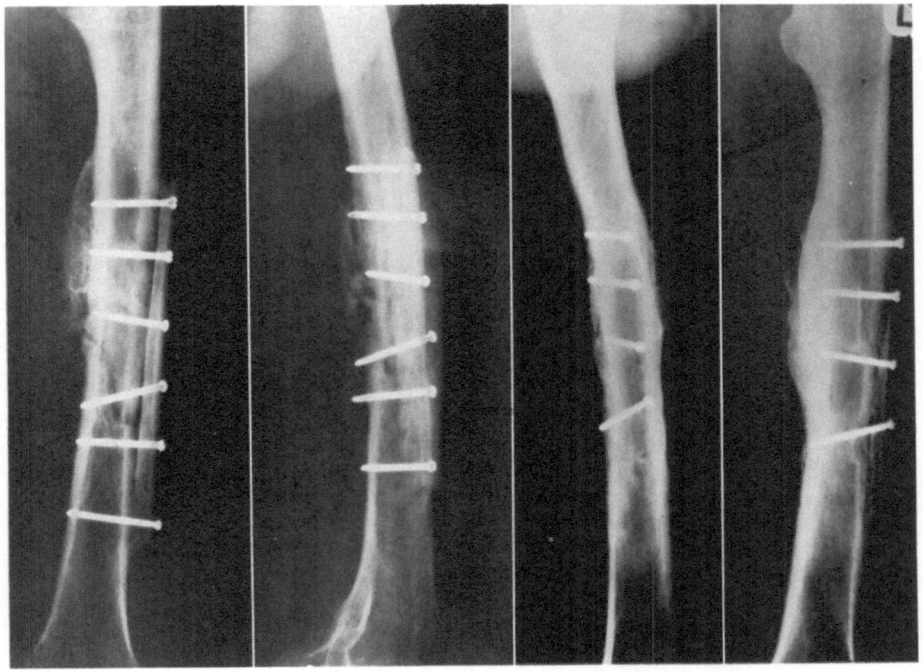

Figure V.2c   Figure V.2d

49

27–6–1969: Patient is quite satisfied with the result. *He has an ache in his left thigh, which radiates down the inner side of the lower leg.*
Occupation: supervisor of assembling central heating installations.
Permanent disability percentage: 45%.
Under the new legislative act, he has bought it off. When standing, the ant. sup. iliac spines were at approximately the same level. The scar, running from the trochanter down the whole length of the outer side of the thigh, and situated at the posterior edge of the vastus lateralis, looked normal. The vastus lateralis muscle was well developed. Femoral axis normal. There was approximately 1 cm shortening, with no contracture of the hip joint as regards flexion and extension. Abduction 20°, adduction 10°, external rotation 10° but very little internal rotation was possible. Knee function normal. No oedema, no varicosities.
During the supporting phase of ambulation, the extension of the right knee was more pronounced than the extension of the left knee. Duration of supporting phase of the left leg was shorter. Standing, the iliac crests were at about the same level, and the left foot had more valgus than the right. Trendelenburg's sign was negative.

Summary: This is an example of a difficult case with *multiple injuries*, in which application of a bone-bank graft led to a very good result.

50

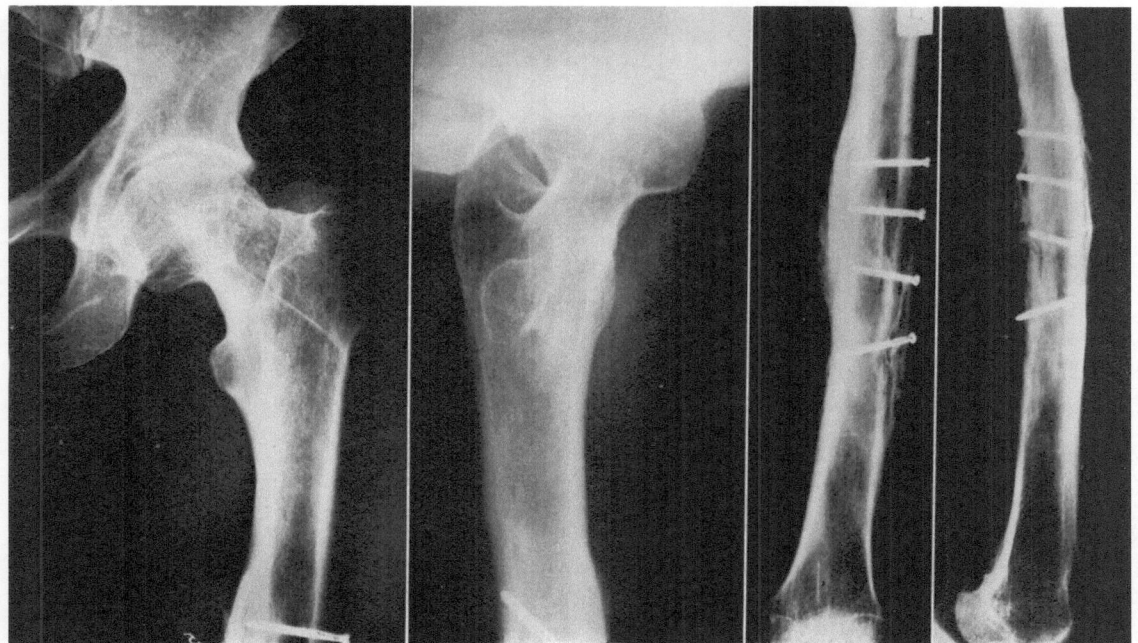

Figure V.2e

Diagnosis: multiple injuries.

Course:

12–2–1962: accident, admitted to Orth. Dept. W.G., concussion, fracture of right femur, compound fracture of left femur, fracture of the pelvis, injury to urethra, fracture of the left tibia and fibula.

13–4–1962: operation: osteosynthesis of the right femur with the aid of a Küntscher nail and homogenous graft.

14–5–1962: same operation on left femur. Post-operative course satisfactory.

6–6–1963: consolidation.

Examination:

13–2–1964: patient, satisfied, is back to work.

Radiographs:

4–4–1962: figure V.3a, unsatisfactory position of the fragments of the *right femur*.

16–4–1962: figure V.3b, right femur post-operative.

6–6–1963: figure V.3c, right femur, Küntscher nail removed, consolidation.

17–4–1962: figure V.3d, left femur, unsatisfactory position of the fragments.

14–5–1962: figure V.3e and V.3f, left femur post-operative.

6–6–1963: figure V.3g, left femur, consolidation in good position.

Summary: A good example of the advantages that are enjoyed by having a bone-bank at one's disposal for solving the problems posed by a patient with multiple injuries.

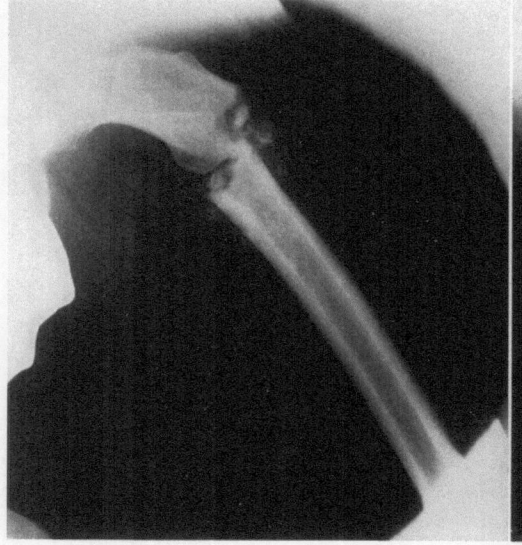 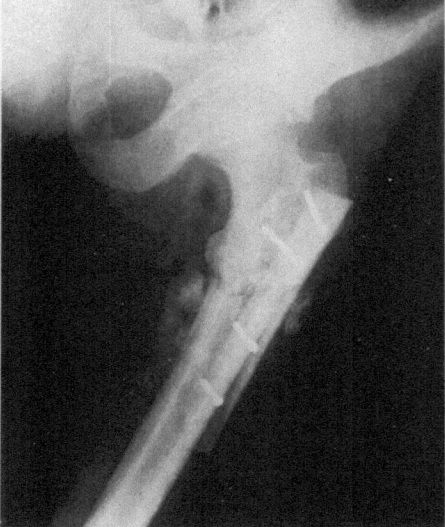 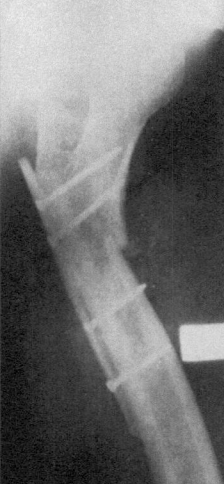

Figure V.3d   Figure V.3e   Figure V.3f

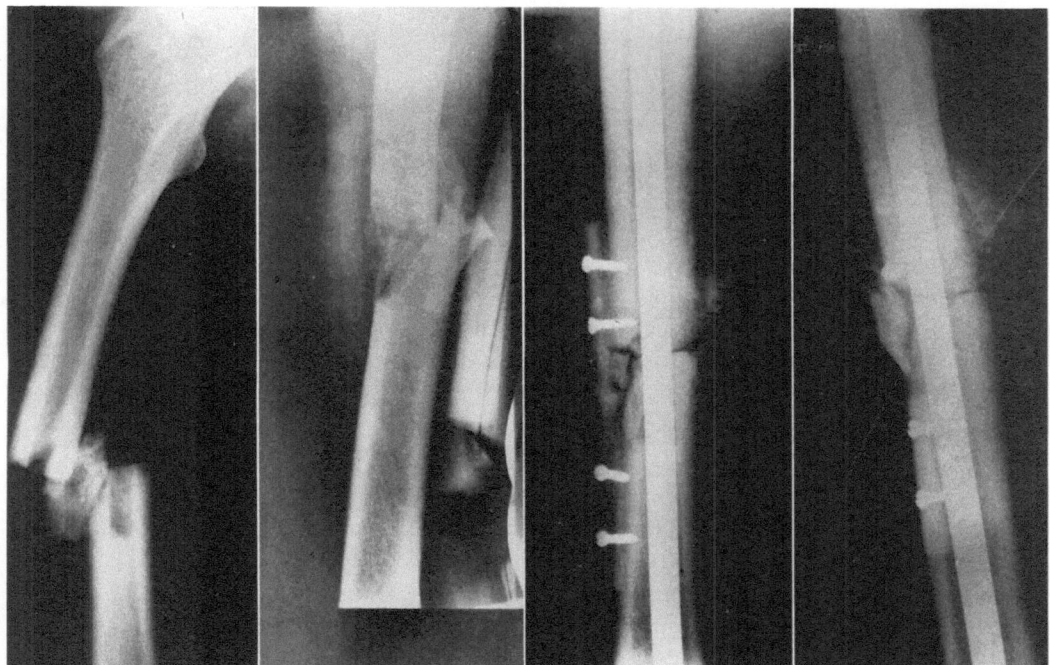

Figure V.3a   Figure V.3b

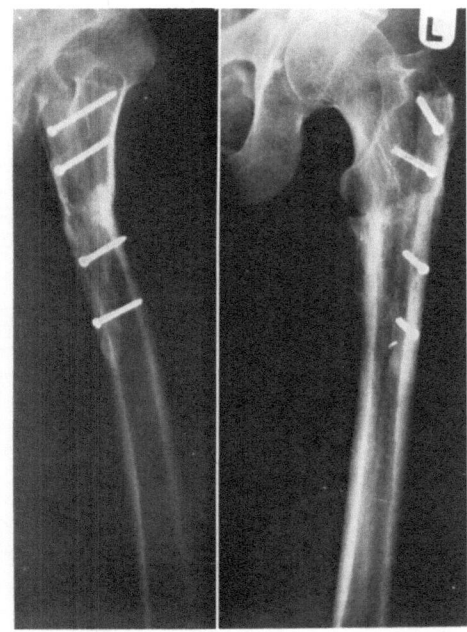

Figure V.3g

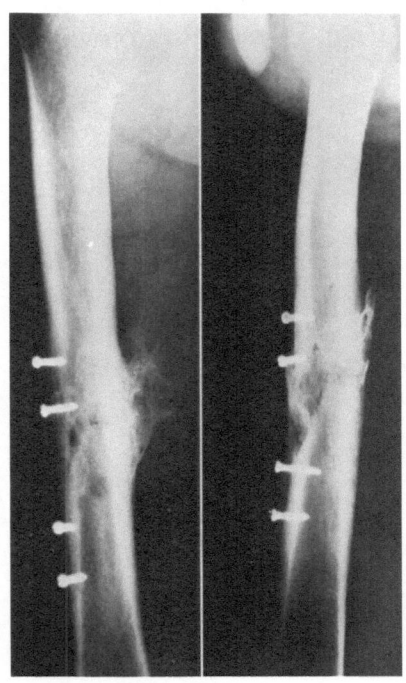

Figure V.3c

Diagnosis: fracture of the left femur.

Course:
18–9–1961:   accident, admitted to Orth. Dept. W.G., fracture of left femur, skeletal traction.
9–10–1961:   unsatisfactory reduction.
10–10–1961:   operation: osteosynthesis with a homogenous graft, balanced suspension and skin traction.
7–11–1961:   transferred to country hospital.
14–12–1961:   fractured graft, varus deformity of the femoral fracture.
15–1–1962:   consolidation, mobilization.

Radiographs:
21–9–1961:   figure V.4a, fracture of the shaft of the left femur with a separate fragment.
10–10–1961:   figure V.4b, post-operative, good position.
15–1–1962:   figure V.4c, fracture consolidated, fracture of the graft.
6–3–1963:   figure V.4d, fracture consolidated with varus deformity.

Summary: This case was registered as a failure because of fracture of the graft. This probably occurred during transport to another hospital.
This observation shows that it is necessary to protect a fracture treated with a homogenous graft from great stresses, and that it is imperative to apply a splint during transport.

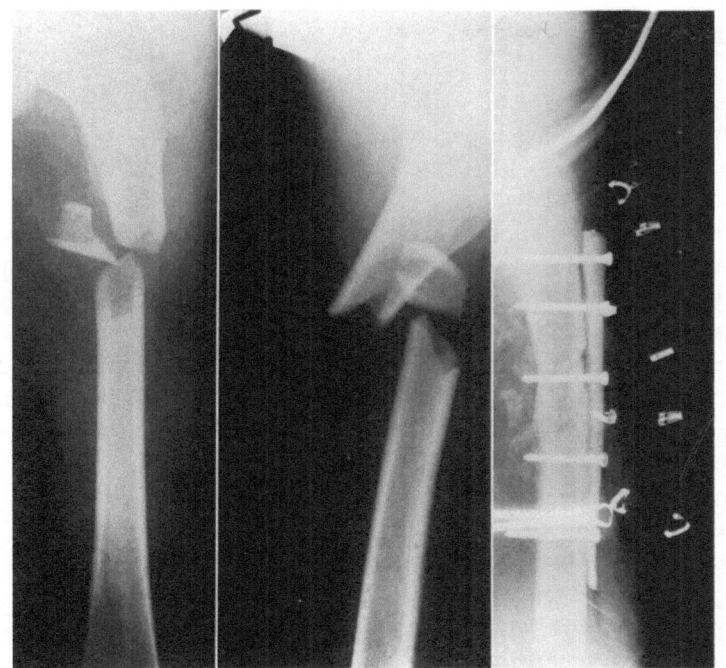

Figure V.4a   Figure V.4b

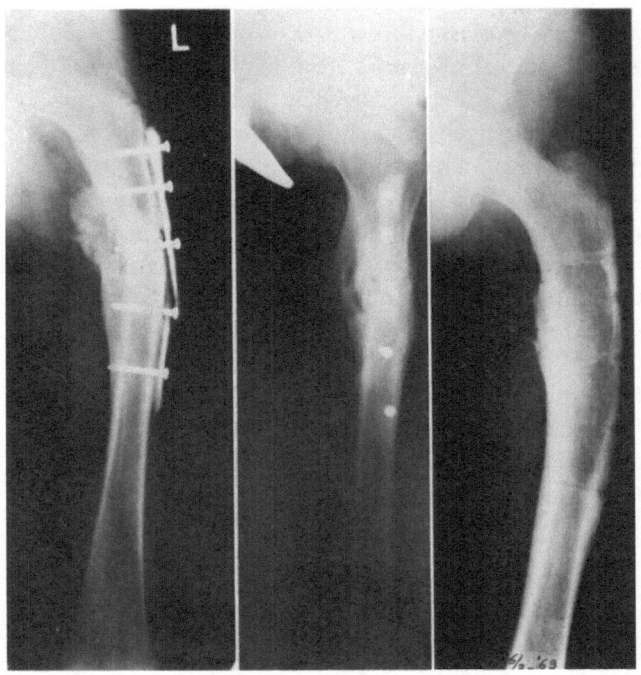

Figure V.4c   Figure V.4d

Diagnosis: multiple fractures, hypersensitivity.

Course:

20–11–1961:   car accident, frontal collision, admitted to Orth. Dept. W. G. with multiple injuries, viz. concussion, facial wounds, fractures of the facial bones, compound fracture of the left ulna, dislocation of the left radial head, fractured ribs, pneumothorax on the left side, fracture of the left femur.

20–11–1961:   operation: suturing of the wounds, anaesthesia with kemital, pethidine, given macrodex, blood transfusions, anti-tetanic serum, anti-gas gangrene serum, tetanus toxoid and during the days following penicillin, streptomycin, tetracycline, luminal, atropine, soneryl.

21–11–1961:   *operation:* drainage of the thorax.

6–12–1961:   skin eruption (caused by drugs?).

8–12–1961:   *operation* by eye-surgeon, reduction of facial fractures.

22–12–1961:   *operation* on the left femur, reduction of the fracture. The Küntscher nail did not provide a sufficient stability, therefore a small homogenous graft was added.

10–1–1962:   *operation* by eye-surgeon.

2–2–1962:   *operation:* resection of left radial head.

19–2–1962:   *operation:* osteosynthesis of left ulna with the aid of a homogenous graft.

27–3–1962:   *operation:* reduction of orbital fracture.

1–2–1963:   *operation* on face by plastic surgeon.

21–3–1963:   *operation* for removal of screws from left femur. After induction with kemital and pethidine profound shock occurred, which could only be reversed with great difficulties. The patient recovered. Further investigation showed that the patient was allergic to penicillin and barbiturates.

22–1–1964:   *operation* because of pseudarthrosis of the left femur. The Küntscher nail was removed and a thick one substituted. The homogenous graft was removed and an autogenous one inserted. Post-operative course was satisfactory without complications.

10–6–1965:   consolidation of the fracture of the femur.

Radiographs:

27–11–1961:   figure V.5a, fracture of left femoral shaft.

22–12–1961:   figure V.5b, post-operative.

12–9–1963:   figure V.5c, pseudarthrosis.

10–6–1965:   figure V.5d, consolidation.

Examination:

30–11–1967:   good form and function of left thigh.

Summary: A male aged 34 with multiple injuries; osteosynthesis of the fracture of the femur with a Küntscher nail and homogenous graft was followed by the development of pseud-

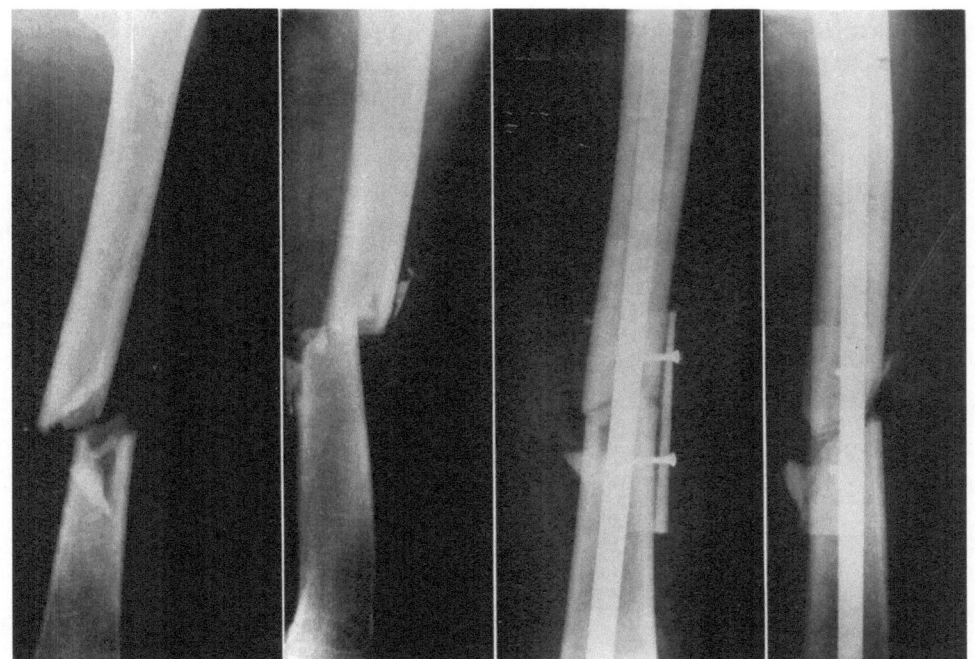

Figure V.5a   Figure V.5b

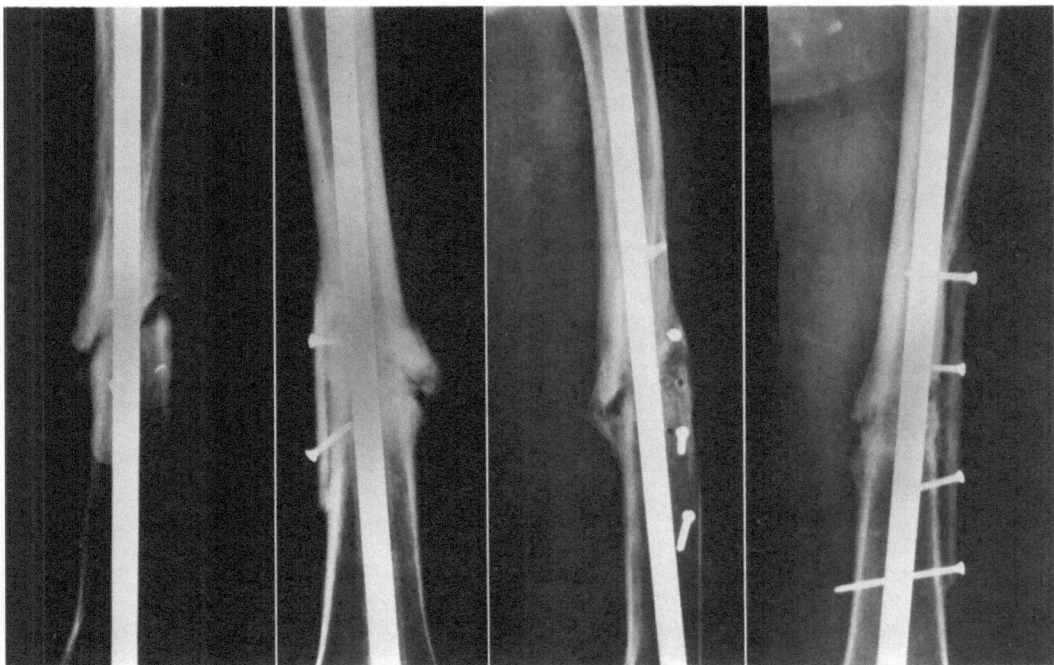

Figure V.5c   Figure V.5d

arthrosis. This failure was caused by *unstable osteosynthesis* due to poor surgical technique. This patient also showed serious manifestations of hypersensitivity. The question arises whether the two successive implantations of homogenous bone may be blamed for this. It should be noted, however, that this patient had ten operations, that for the induction of anaesthesia in each of these ten operations barbiturates were used, that penicilline and other antibiotics were also administered, and that a skin eruption (often first manifestation of hypersensitivity) occurred *before* the first implantation of bone graft. It is therefore not plausible that the homogenous bone tissue was responsible for the hypersensitivity.

There was hypersensitivity to penicillin and barbiturates. On 1–5–1969 extraction of Küntscher nail and the dist. screw was performed under anaesthesia without complication. Penicillin and barbiturates were not used.

PATIENT V.6, MALE, BORN 27–1–1946

Diagnosis: fracture of the left femur.

Course:

26–8–1964: motor-cycle accident, multiple injuries, including a fracture of the left femur.

15–9–1964: operation: osteosynthesis of femoral fracture with a *homogenous* bone graft.

14–1–1965: walking with elbow crutches.

25–3–1965: operation: occipito-cervical (C$_1$, C$_2$, C$_3$) fusion performed, because of fracture of the odontoid proces, with autogenous tibial graft.

19–2–1968: *refracture of left femur sustained following slight trauma.*

27–2–1968: operation: exposure of left femoral shaft, the graft was firmly united to the femur, and had to be removed with a hammer and chisel. The graft appeared to have undergone complete reconstruction at its extremities, but *the central part, i.e. the part at the level of the fracture, was dead and not fixed to the femur; the fracture was a new, recent fracture. This fracture was now stabilized with an autogenous graft from the right tibia.*

1–10–1968: consolidation.

Radiographs:

26–8–1964: figure V.6a, fracture of femur with separate triangular fragment.

18–9–1964: figure V.6b, post-operative, osteosynthesis with homogenous graft.

12–2–1965: figure V.6c, extensive bridging by callus on medial side.

Continuation on page 60

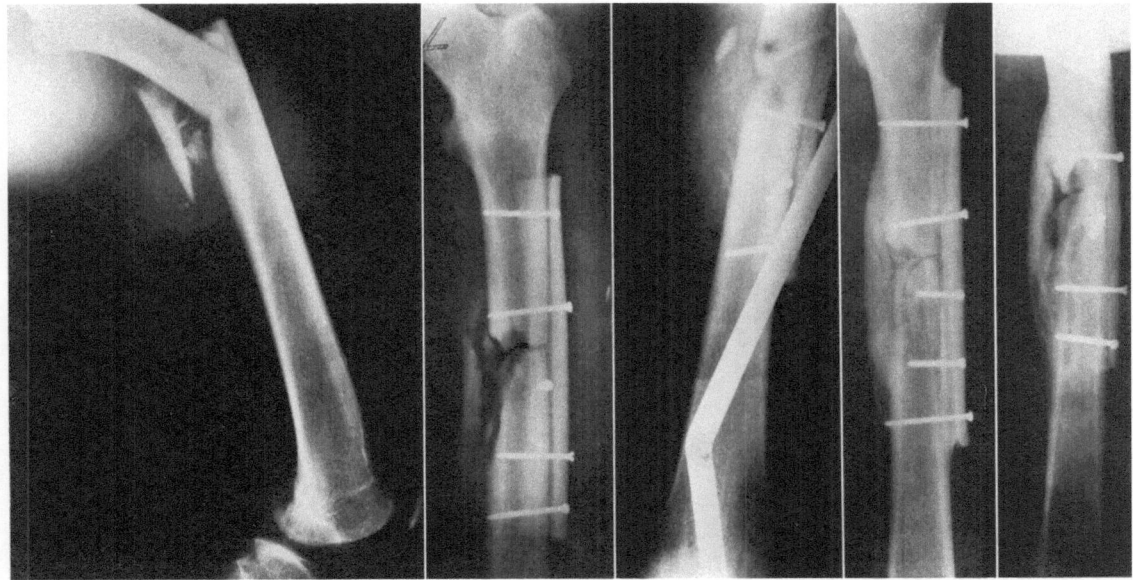

Figure V.6a   Figure V.6b   Figure V.6c

30–9–1965:	figure V.6d, consolidation.
18–1–1968:	figure V.6e, fracture consolidated, part of the graft firmly united to femur – structurally assimilated with femoral shaft.
20–2–1968:	figure V.6f, refracture at the level of the central screw, but at a different level from the previous fracture – in fragment there was probably no shaft building.
1–3–1968:	figure V.6g, post-operative.
16–10–1968:	figure V.6h, consolidation.

Summary: Case of osteosynthesis of a fractured femur in a male aged 18, which healed well, but a refracture occurred 3 years later. Probably there was no shaft structure. Microscopical examination of the graft was performed.

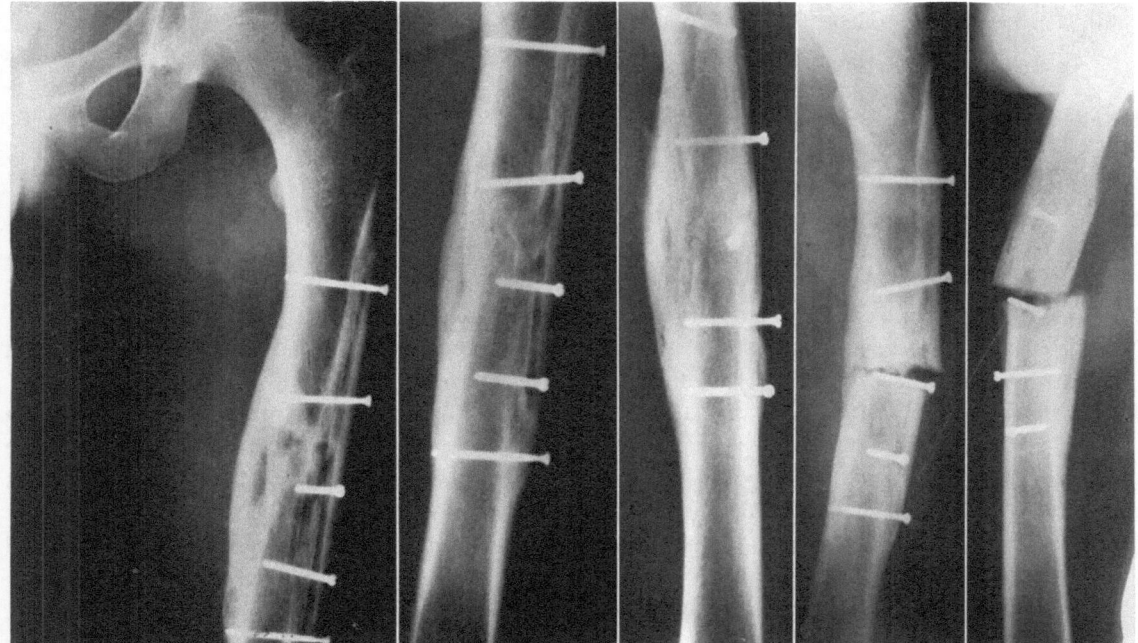

Figure V.6d   Figure V.6e   Figure V.6f

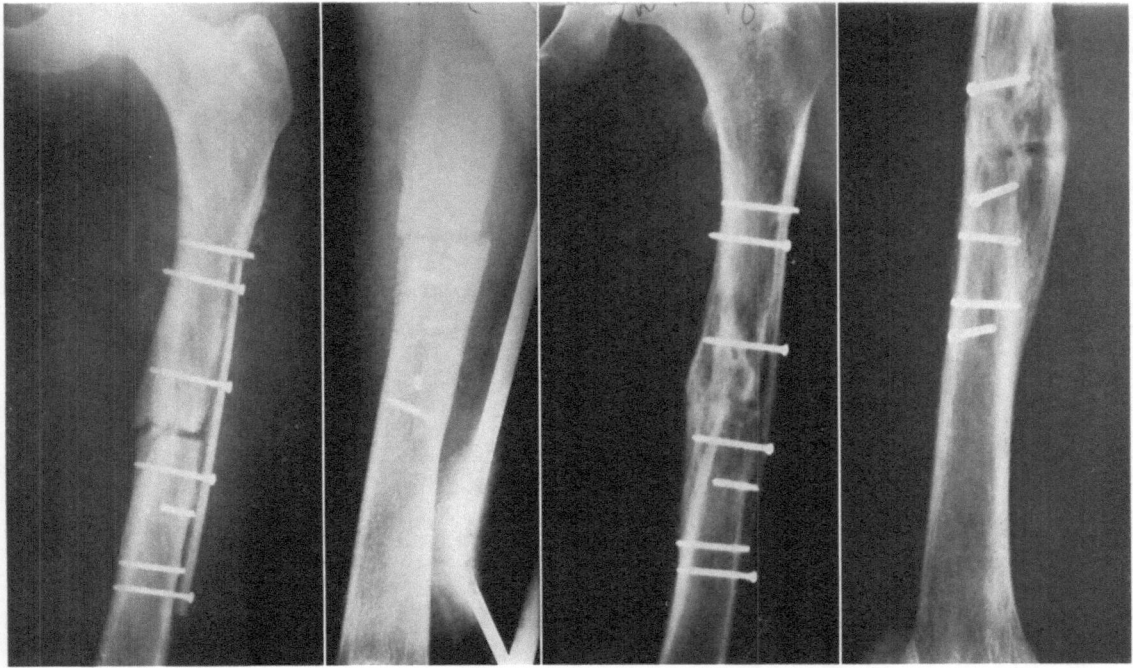

Figure V.6g   Figure V.6h

61

Diagnosis: fracture of the right femur.

Course:

15–1–1963:   fall on the slippery pavement, admitted to Orth. Dept. W.G.; fracture of right femur.

16–1–1963:   operation: osteosynthesis of the fracture of the right femur with a homogenous graft. Post-operative course satisfactory, primary healing.

14–8–1963:   fracture consolidated, patient already mobilized.

29–9–1964:   was pushed in the street, fell, and again sustained a fracture of the right femur, but this was a different type of fracture to the first one.

8–10–1964:   re-operation: anaesthesia, patient positioned on his side, an incision was made along the scar of the previous operation, with exposure of the fractured fragments. There was a recent fracture at the level of one of the screws. The bone-bank graft which was applied in 16–1–1963 showed satisfactory bony union with the femur, the graft was white and did not contain bloodvessels. The heads of the screws projected beyond the level of the graft. The screws were removed, a vitallium Küntscher nail, 40 cm long and 10 mm wide, was inserted. The position of the fragments was satisfactory, but the fracture was not quite stable. *A different bone-bank graft from a different donor was now fixed to the fractured fragments with short screws.* Then the fracture was quite stable. The wound was closed in layers.
X-ray check: good position achieved.

8–3–1965:   patient already mobilized.

21–4–1965:   walks well without crutches.

Examination: No further information was available.

Radiographs:

16–1–1963:   figure V.7a, fracture of the right femur.

17–1–1963:   figure V.7b, post-operative.

14–8–1963:   figure V.7c and figure V.7d, consolidated in good position.

2–10–1964:   figure V.7e, fractured again, at a different level.

8–10–1964:   figure V.7f, post-operative.

4–2–1965:   figure V.7g, consolidation.

Summary: A male aged 87 who twice sustained a fracture of the femur which was twice successfully treated with a bone-bank graft. This is the oldest patient in our series. A bone-bank graft has great advantages for these very old people.

Indication for osteosynthesis:
An old man who presents problems in nursing. One of the femoral fragments was pointed and projected into the groin; thus there was the risk of injury to the great vessels.

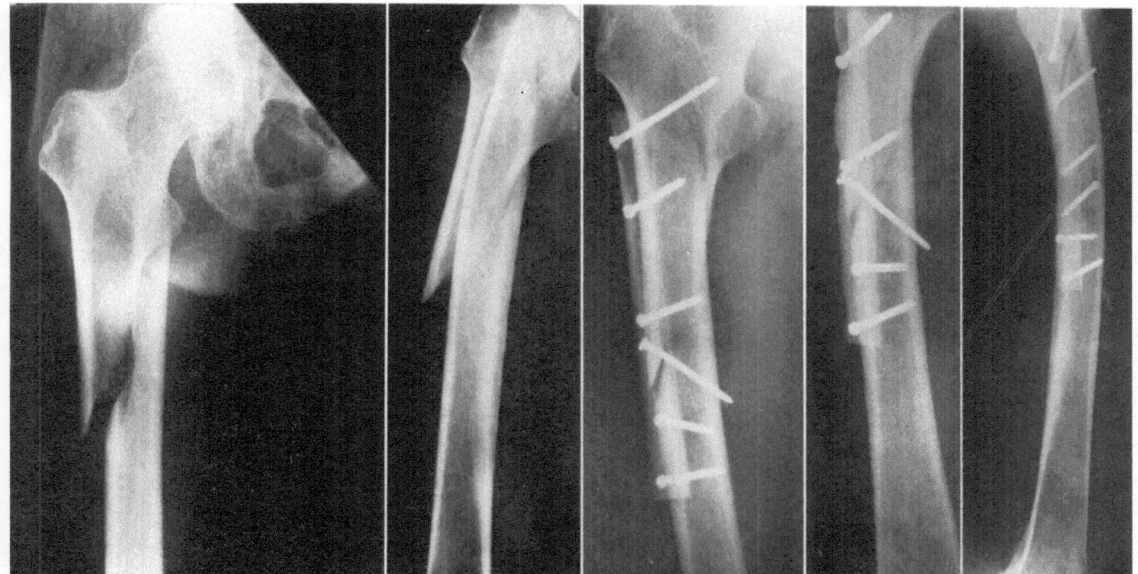

Figure V.7a   Figure V.7b   Figure V.7c   Figure V.7d

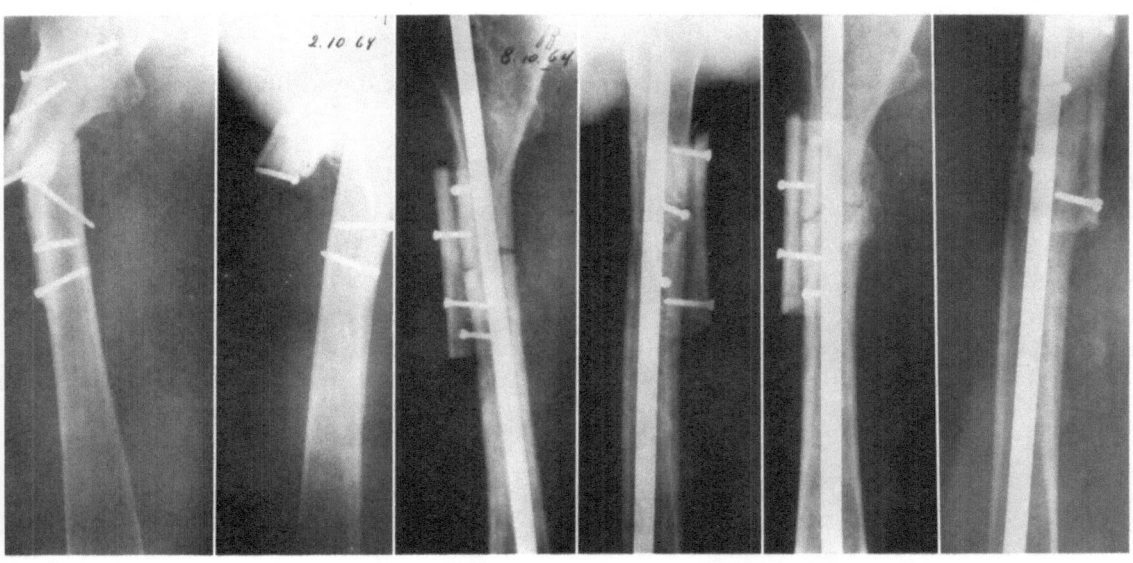

Figure V.7e   Figure V.7f   Figure V.7g

Diagnosis: pseudarthrosis of the femur.

Previous history:
20–10–1953:   accident, fracture of the left femur and a Y-shaped fracture of tibial condyles.
5–11–1953:   osteosynthesis of the femur with a Küntscher nail and circular wiring. Osteosynthesis of tibial condyles.

Course: The patient was first seen by us in January 1954. There was *suppuration* along the track of the skeletal traction pin through the distal end of the left femur, pressure sores near the fibular head and on the heel, paralysis of the peroneal nerve, and dystrophy of the left leg.
Our treatment consisted of removal of the skeletal traction, application of balanced skin traction, attention to the pressure sores and active excercises.
14–10–1955:   the function of the extremity had improved. A pseudarthrosis had developed and the metal used for the osteosynthesis was removed.
9–3–1956:   operation of the left thigh, treatment of the pseudarthrosis and fixation with a homogenous graft. After-treatment in bed with balanced suspension and skin-traction.
17–10–1956:   healing.
1–1–1971:   good condition.

Examination:
29–11–1968:   intermittantly the inflammation flares up along the track caused by the skeletal traction, otherwise the patient is quite well.

Radiographs:
14–10–1955:   figure V.8a, left femur, pseudarthrosis.
24–4–1956:   figure V.8b, 6 weeks post-operative.
13–2–1957:   figure V.8c, consolidation.

Summary: Case of an extremely difficult pseudarthrosis, which healed after fixation with a homogenous graft. Indication against the use of a Küntscher nail was *the infection caused by skeletal traction during first treatment*.

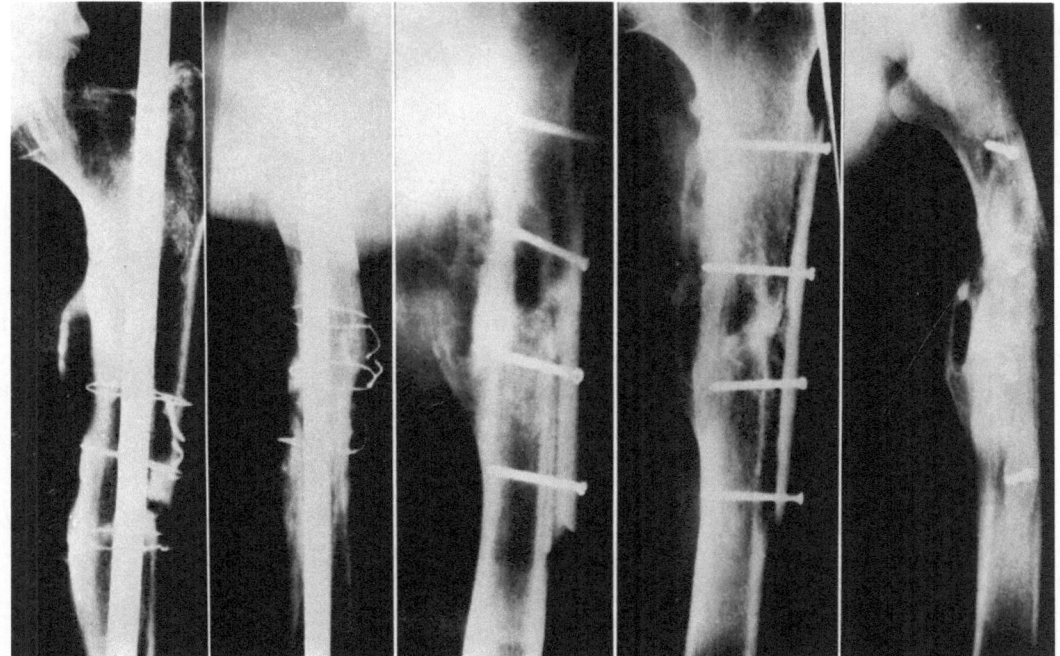

Figure V.8a   Figure V.8b   Figure V.8c

Diagnosis: pseudarthrosis of the right humerus.

Previous history:

1948:	accident, fracture of humerus.
1949:	operation, osteosynthesis with a Küntscher nail, pseudarthrosis developed.
1950:	operation, osteosynthesis with metal plate and autogenous bone, again no bony union.
11–8–1955:	refracture through the old pseudarthrosis, operation with Küntscher nail and autogenous bone chips, pseudarthrosis developed. From 1956 on the patient, at the request of the Social Insurance Service (S.V.B.), came under our medical care. He still had a pseudarthrosis.

Course:

13–4–1956:	operation: homogenous graft applied to the humerus, *with autogenous cancellous bone chips from the iliac crest*, after-treatment with abduction splint.
13–11–1956:	there was now a bony consolidation of the humerus.
15–4–1958:	on examination good result obtained.

Radiographs:

5–1–1956:	figure V.9a and figure V.9b, pseudarthrosis of humerus.
11–9–1956:	figure V.9c, post-operative.
13–11–1956:	figure V.9d, consolidation.
15–4–1958:	figure V.9e, last X-ray.

Summary: Male aged 55 with pseudarthrosis of the right humerus which had been present for 8 years, and which had already been treated elsewhere three times by surgery without success. Consolidation in 7 months after treatment with a *homogenous graft*.

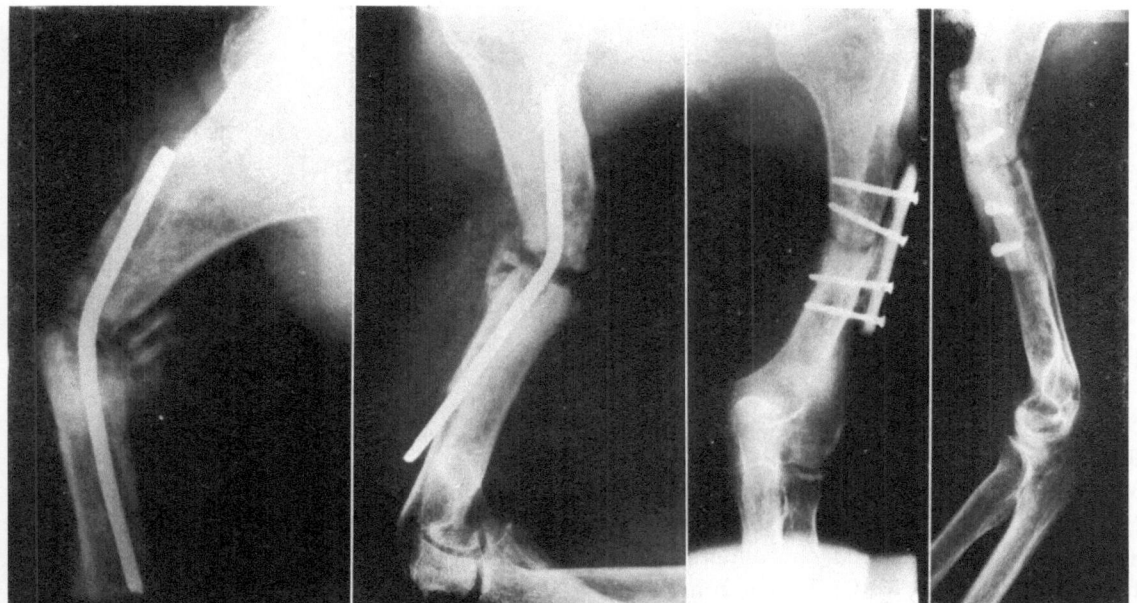

Figure V.9a   Figure V.9b   Figure V.9c

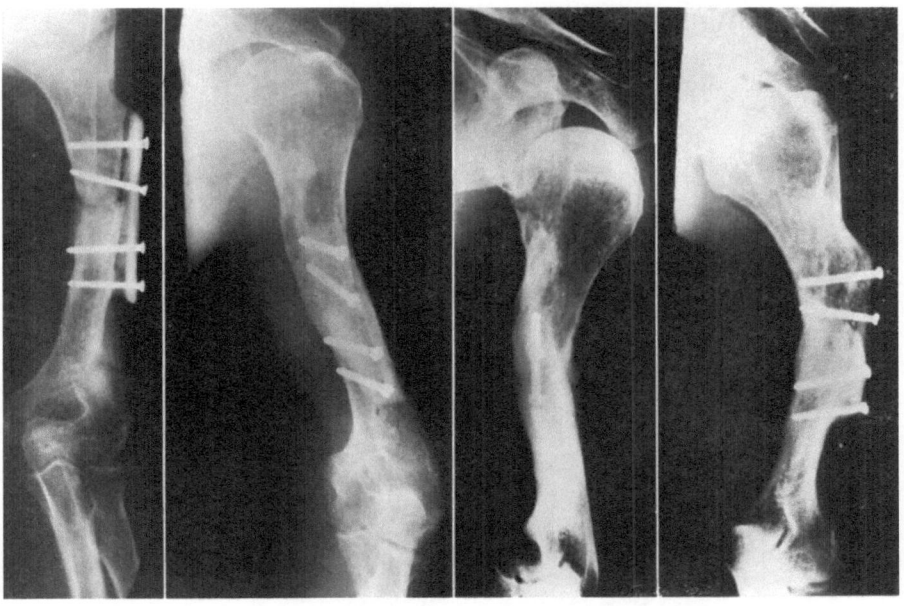

Figure V.9d   Figure V.9e

67

Previous history: recorded osteomyelitis of the left tibia at the age of 6, which led to pseudarthrosis; plastic repair with autogenous graft. This failed.

Course:

16–7–1961: admitted to Orth. Dept. W.G. with pseudarthrosis of the left tibia and dystrophy of the bone and soft tissues; rehabilitation was instituted as a preliminary treatment.

6–2–1962: operation: resection of the pseudarthrosis, plastic repair with 2 homogenous bone grafts. Satisfactory course, good result.

1–9–1964: re-operation because of a zone of Looser in the tibia, the bone grafts inserted in 1962, appeared to have been completely assimilated. Again application of homogenous bone graft. Satisfactory course, good result.

Radiographs:

30–1–1962: figure V.10a and 10b, pseudarthrosis of left tibia, marked atrophy of tibia and fibula.

6–2–1962: figure V.10c, post-operative.

9–5–1963: figure V.10d, consolidation.

13–8–1964: figure V.10e, Looser-zone.

1–9–1964: figure V.10f, post-operative.

30–5–1969: figure V.10g, consolidation with homogenous graft.

Summary: Case of pseudarthrosis in thin atrophic bone; grafting with autogenous bone had failed, success with a double homogenous graft. *After 2½ years Looser's zone successfully treated by again using a homogenous graft.*

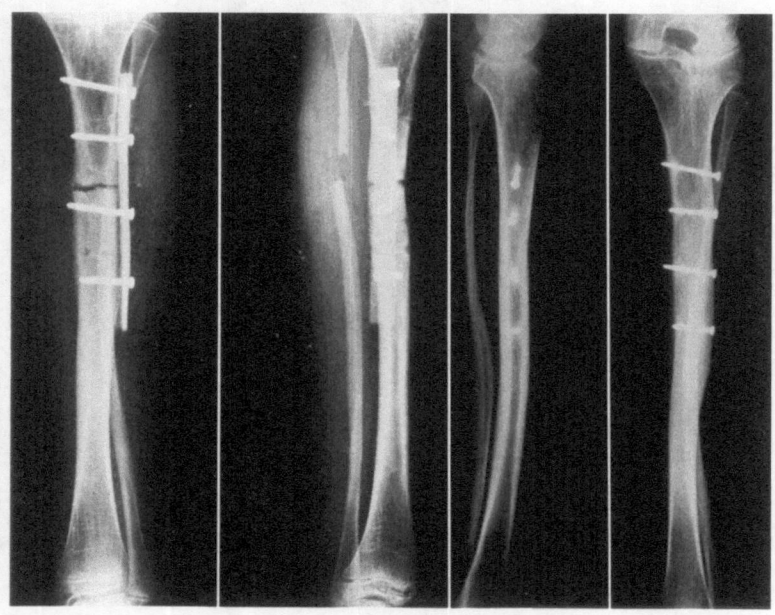

Figure V.10f   Figure V.10g

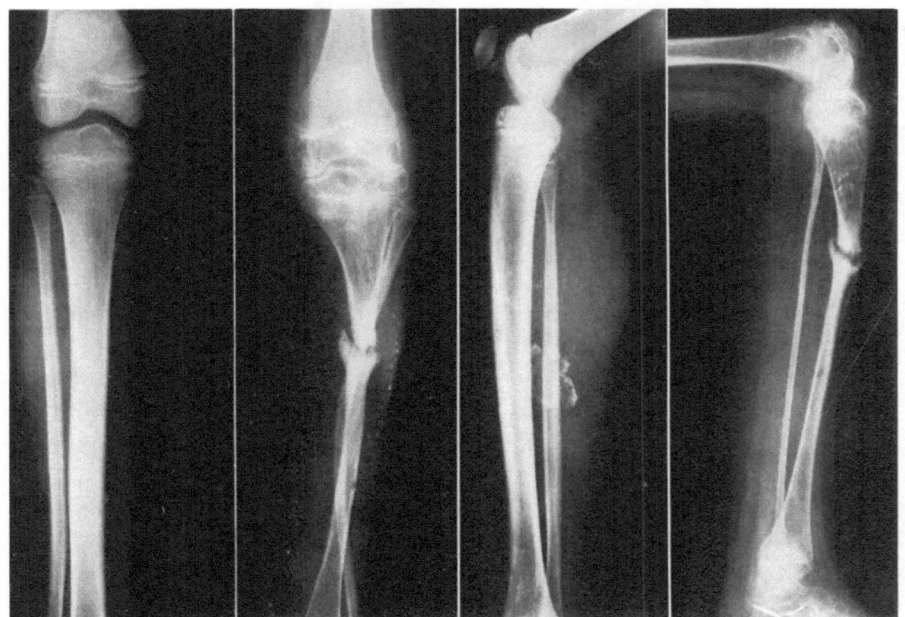

Figure V.10a   Figure V.10b

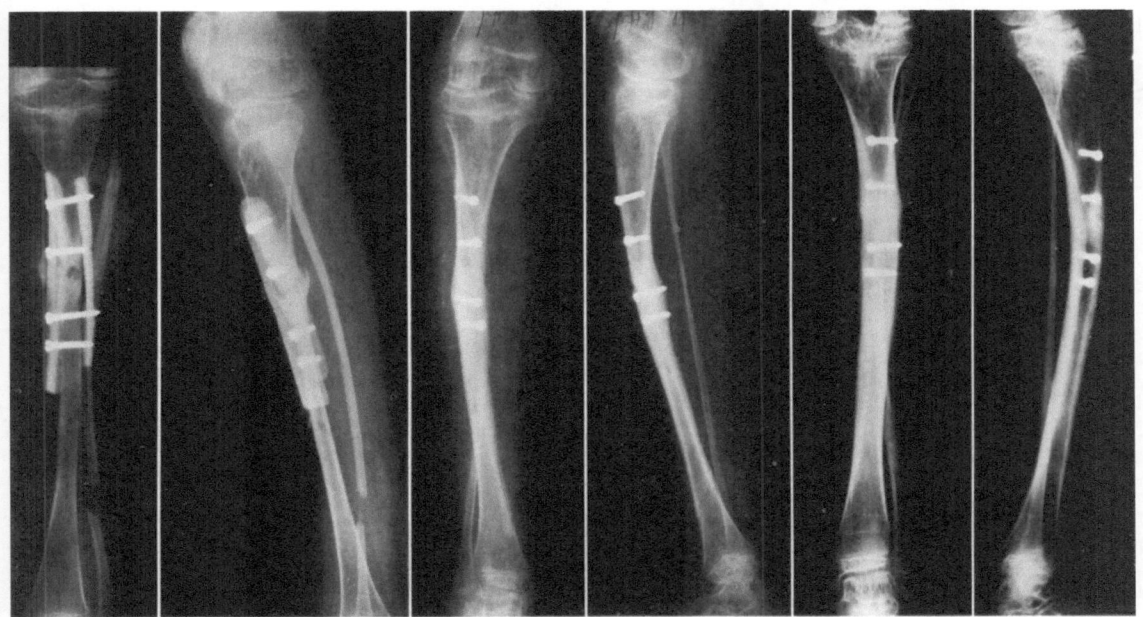

Figure V.10c   Figure V.10d   Figure V.10e

Previous history:

| 1950: | sarcoma of the left femur, treated by intensive X-ray therapy, tumour healed! |
| 1955: | spontaneous fracture of the left femur resulting in pseudarthrosis. |

Course:

22–12–1955:	admitted to Orth. Dept. W.G. because of pseudarthrosis of left femur with marked atrophy of bone, muscular tissue and skin.
1955–1957:	several skin grafting operations to obtain good skin at the level of the fracture (figure V.11a).
29–9–1958:	pseudarthrosis operation with homogenous graft.
14–2–1959:	mobilized in a Thomas splint.
10–3–1960:	consolidation of the fracture.
Dec. 1970:	perfect condition.

Examination:

| 19–4–1968: | patient in good condition, left leg stable, has extension-appliance to compensate for the shortening of the left leg. |

Radiographs:

12–12–1957:	figure V.11b and figure V.11c, pseudarthrosis of the left femur.
24–12–1958:	figure V.11d and figure V.11e, post-operative.
19–4–1968:	figure V.11f and figure V.11g, consolidated fracture, reconstruction of shaft.

Summary: Here we have a boy treated by massive X-ray therapy because of a sarcoma of the left femur. The X-ray therapy caused a pathological fracture with marked atrophy of soft tissues. After skin grafting and bone grafting with a homogenous graft, the fracture united. Last X-ray, 1968, showed structural consolidation. *Good example of the value of the homogenous graft.*

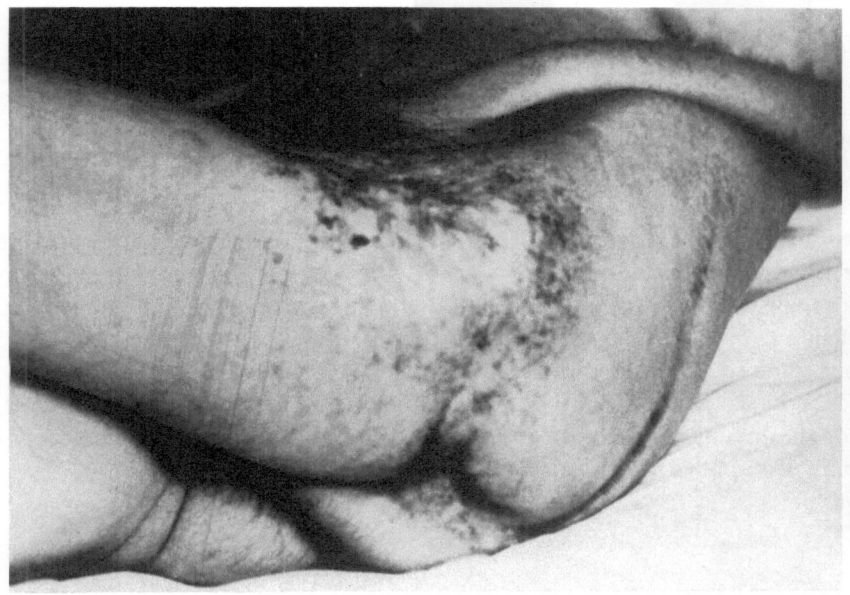

Figure V.11a

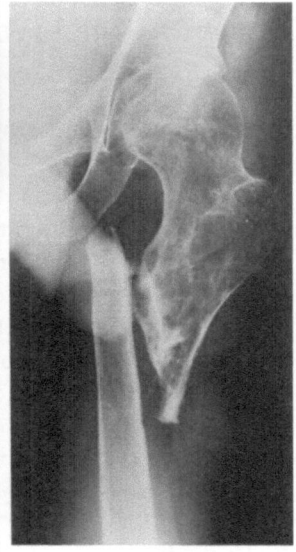

Figure V.11b

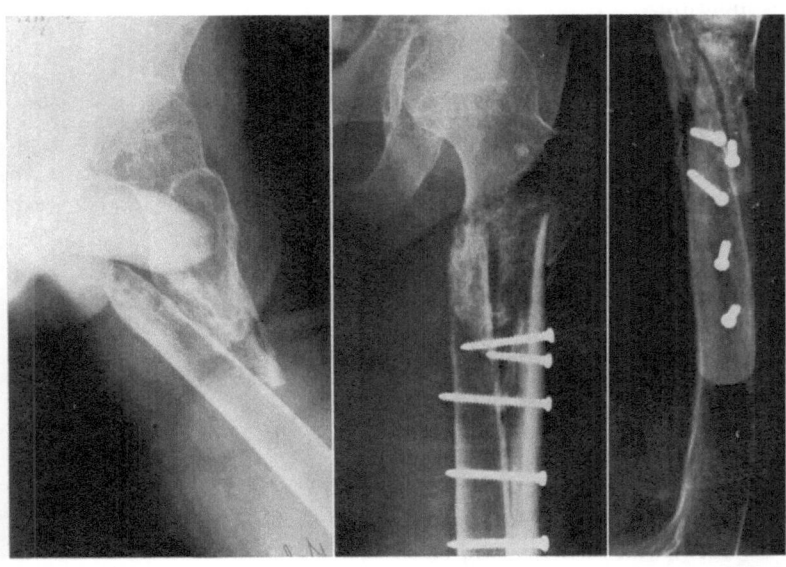

Figure V.11c   Figure V.11d   Figure V.11e   Figure V.11f   Figure V.11g

71

Diagnosis: pseudarthrosis of the left humerus.

Course:

1957:   admitted to S.V.B. (Social Insurance Service) Dept. of the Burgerziekenhuis, because of pseudarthrosis of the left humerus.

1–11–1957:   operation: repair with homogenous bone graft, after-treatment with abduction splint.

25–2–1958:   removal of splint.

6–5–1958:   spontaneous fracture, which did not heal.

30–1–1959:   operation: there was a pseudarthrosis of the humerus and a fracture of the graft, resection of the pseudarthrosis, osteosynthesis with autogenous bone graft. An abduction splint was applied afterwards.

27–10–1959:   bony union.

Radiographs:

1–10–1957:   figure V.12a, pseudarthrosis of left humerus.

1–11–1957:   figure V.12b, post-operative.

6–5–1958:   figure V.12c, fracture of humerus and fracture of graft.

27–10–1959:   figure V.12d, consolidation.

                figure V.12e, macroscopic section of the area: humeral shaft-graft.

Summary: Case of a pseudarthrosis of the humerus in a male aged 41, which was treated with a homogenous graft; 6 months after the operation refracture occurred which again gave rise to pseudarthrosis. *There was bony union 9 months after repair with an autogenous graft.* The specimen obtained at the second operation was examined, it appeared that the graft had good bony union with the underlying humerus, but that the graft, at the site of the fracture which was examined microscopically, had only partly been reconstructed.

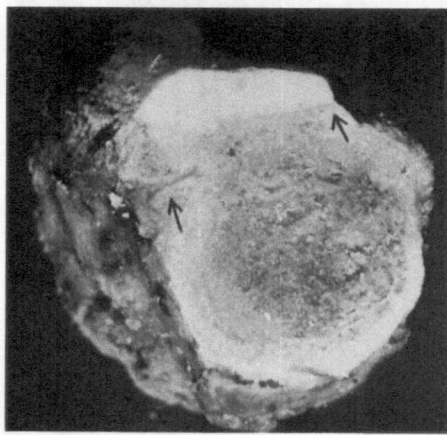

Figure V.12e

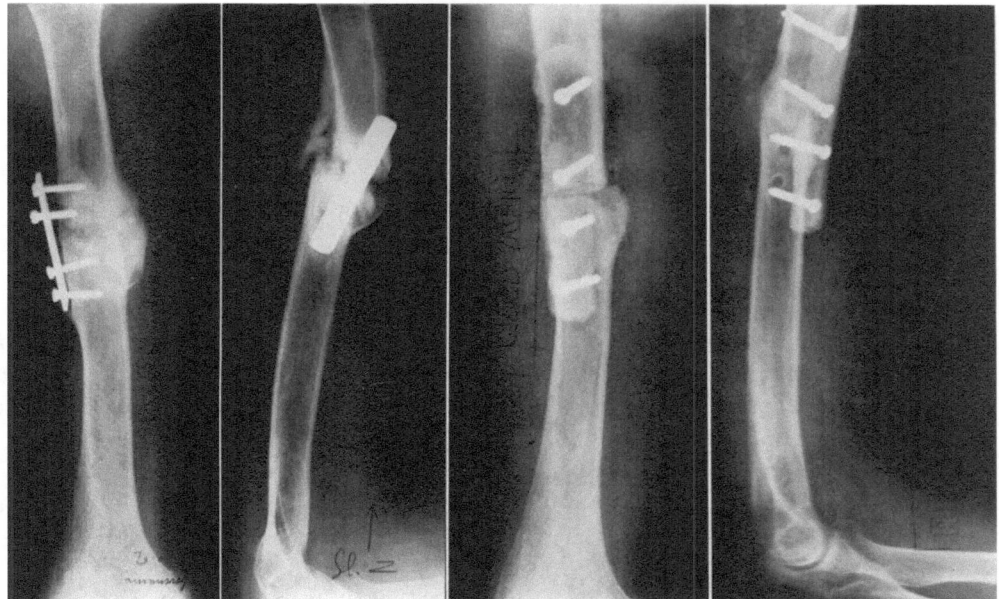

Figure V.12a   Figure V.12b

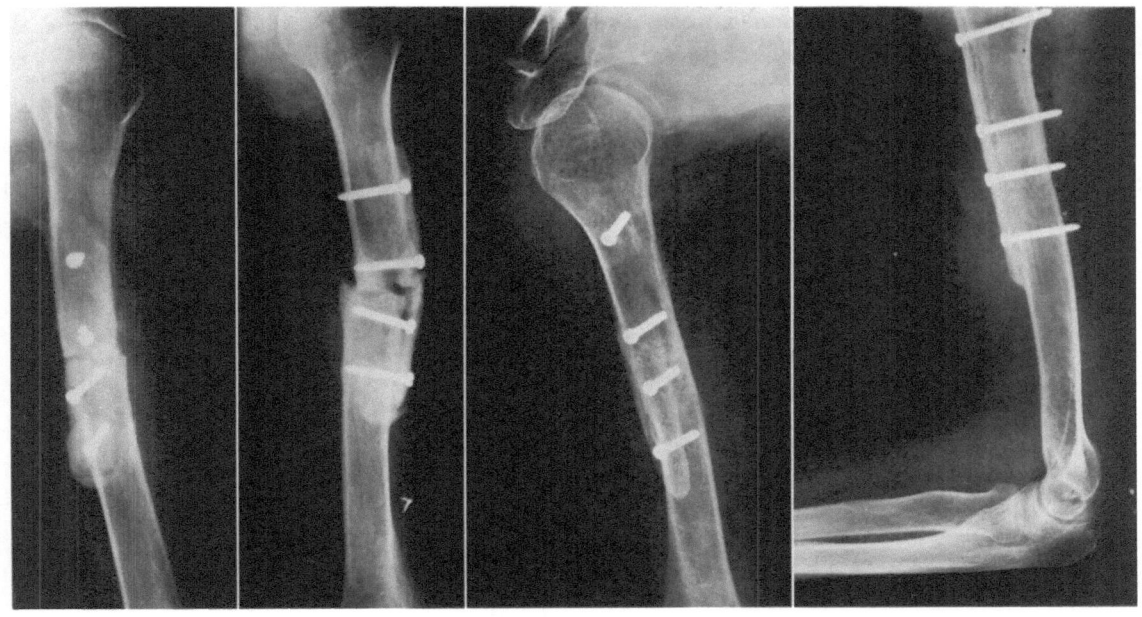

Figure V.12c   Figure V.12d

Previous history:

involved in a car-accident 23–10–1965, compound fracture of the left upper arm, osteosynthesis using a Lane plate and screws, pseudarthrosis developed.

Course:

24–11–1966: admitted to Orth. Dept. W.G. because of pseudarthrosis.

8–12–1966: operation on left upper arm, removal of plate and screws, osteosynthesis *with homogenous graft plus additional strip of autogenous bone from the iliac crest* arranged alongside the fracture. Post-operative course was satisfactory, primary healing occurred. After-treatment with a thoraco-brachial plaster cast.

5–6–1967: plaster removed, consolidation.

April 1968: re-vaccinated against small-pox on the right upper arm. No illness at all because of this, but 3 weeks later the left upper arm became swollen and painful, the scar red, the temperature 39°9 C. This lasted for 2–3 days, after which this reaction quickly subsided.

Examination:

25–10–1968: the patient has no complaints and is very satisfied; good form and function of left upper arm.

Radiographs:

28–11–1966: figure V.13a, pseudarthrosis of left humerus.

8–12–1966: figure V.13b, post-operative.

30–7–1967: figure V.13c, consolidation of the fracture.

28–10–1968: figure V.13d, bony union of graft with underlying humerus.

Summary: Pseudarthrosis of the left upper arm occurring in a young woman successfully treated with a bone-bank graft plus additional strips of autogenous bone. 3 weeks after re-vaccination against small-pox a reaction occurred in the operated arm.

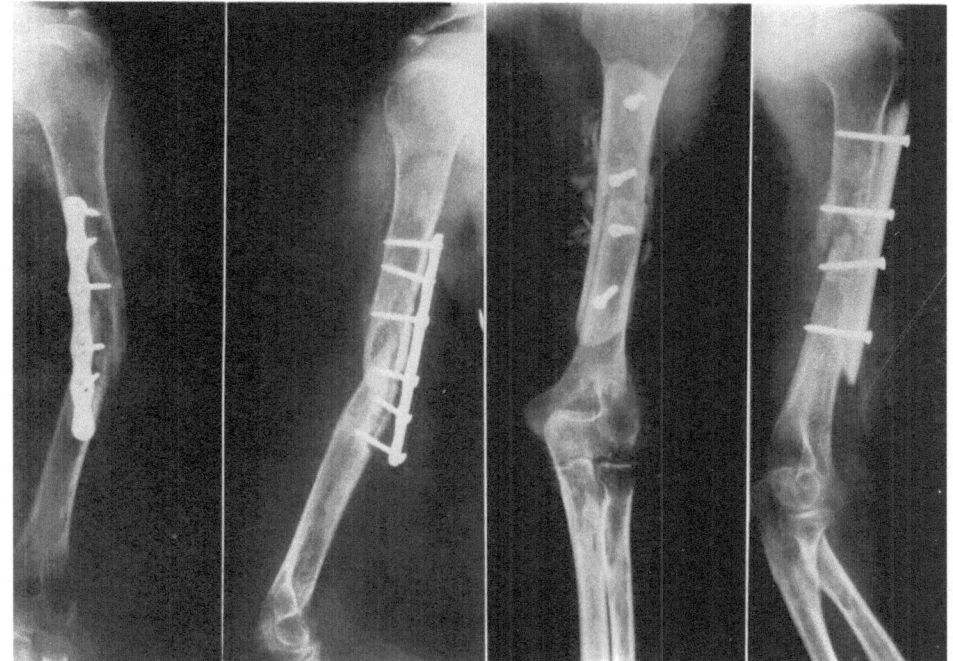

Figure V.13a   Figure V.13b

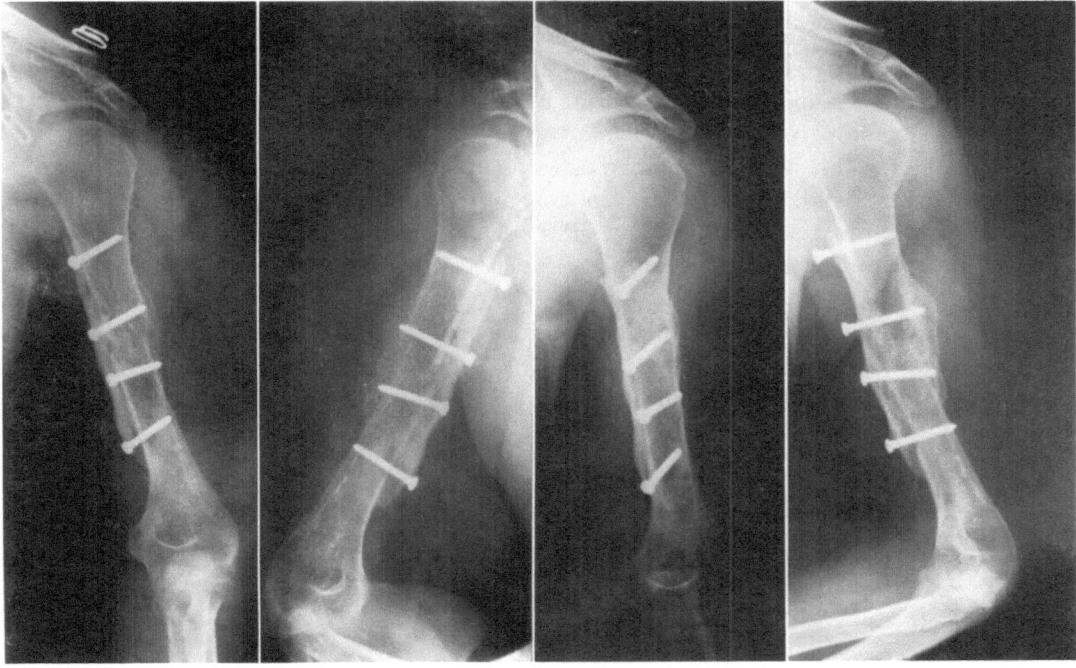

Figure V.13c   Figure V.13d

75

PATIENT V.14, MALE, BORN 7–1–1920

Diagnosis: tuberculous arthritis of the left hip.

Previous history:

1930:   tuberculous arthritis of the hip.
1940:   arthrodesis of the left hip which failed.

Course:
13–3–1956:   admitted to Orth. Dept. W.G. because of increasing pain and instability of the left hip; movement was still possible and an adduction deformity was present. Indication for operation: fibrous ankylosis of the hip joint following tuberculous arthritis.
19–3–1956:   operation carried out on the left hip, a hole was drilled from the major trochanter via the neck of the femur through the joint into the pelvis, and a *homogenous graft* was driven into the hole; and for the correction of the deformity *an intertrochanteric osteotomy* was performed; after-treatment was in a hip plaster spica.
13–12–1956: arthrodesis clinically sound.

Examination:
27–11–1967: patient is complaining of back ache. However, the hip is satisfactory, a bony ankylosis has been obtained.

Radiographs:
20–1–1956:   figure V.14a, pelvis: considerable deformity of the left hip joint; joint space still present.
19–3–1956:   figure (V.14b, X-ray taken during operation with drills in direction of graft (sp.) and osteotomy (o.t.).
13–12–1956: figure V.14c, left hip, graft and osteotomy well visible.
27–11–1967: figure V.14d, left hip, bony ankylosis, joint space has disappeared, continuity of the bone trabeculae, outline of the graft onluy faintly visible. Healing of tuberculosis.
             bone trabeculae, outline of the graft only faintly visible. Healing of tuberculosis.

Summary: Case of intra-articular arthrodesis of the hip, which resulted in a solid bony ankylosis, *strongly suggestive of osteogenic activity of the graft* applied. This was combined with an osteotomy for the correction of the adduction deformity, without osteosynthesis.

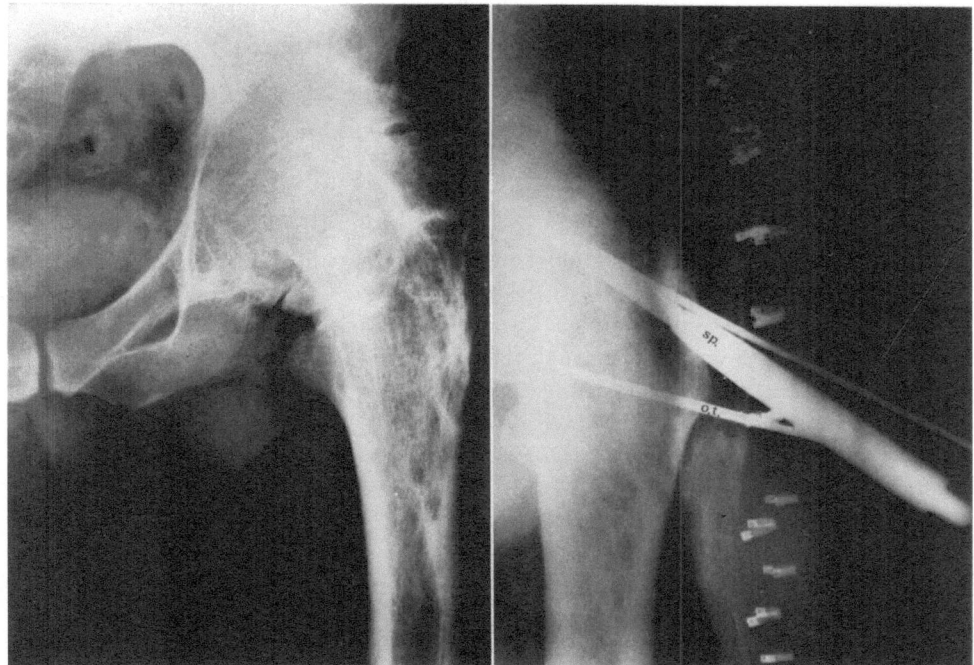

Figure V.14a   Figure V.14b

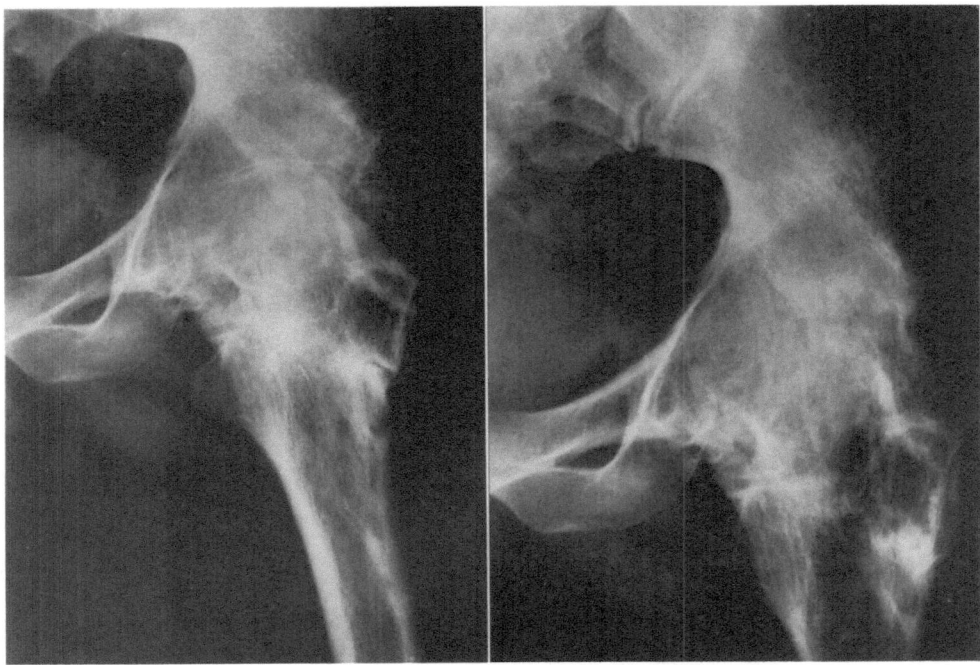

Figure V.14c   Figure V.14d

Diagnosis: paralysis of the right shoulder after poliomyelitis.

Course:
4–12–1964:   admitted to Orth. Dept. W.G.
21–12–1964:   operation on the right shoulder joint, cartilage removed from the humeral head and glenoid cavity, roughening of the caudal surface of acromion, the head positioned in the angle between glenoid cavity and acromion, and there fixed with a homogenous graft which was driven through the acromion into the humeral head. After-treatment in thoraco-branchial plaster.
16–6–1965:   plaster removed, arthrodesis clinically sound.

Examination:
7–4–1966:   patient very satisfied, arthrodesis good.

Radiographs:
10–12–1964:   figure V.15a, right shoulder before operation.
22–12–1964:   figure V.15b, post-operative with graft in situ.
16–9–1965:   figure V.15c, sound arthorodesis with bony union between humeral head and glenoid and between humeral head and acromion; outline of the graft very vague.

Summary: Case of a successful arthrodesis of the shoulder joint with complete assimilation of the graft.

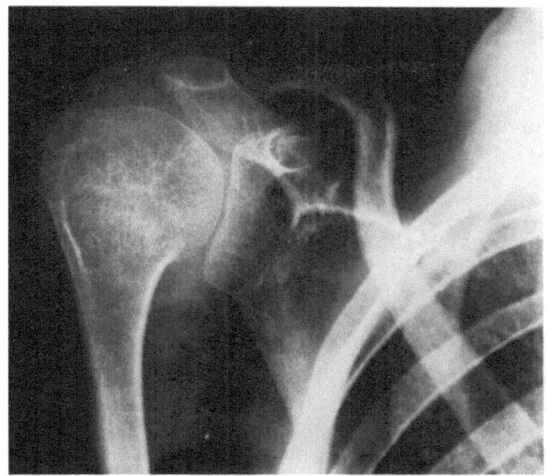

Figure V.15a

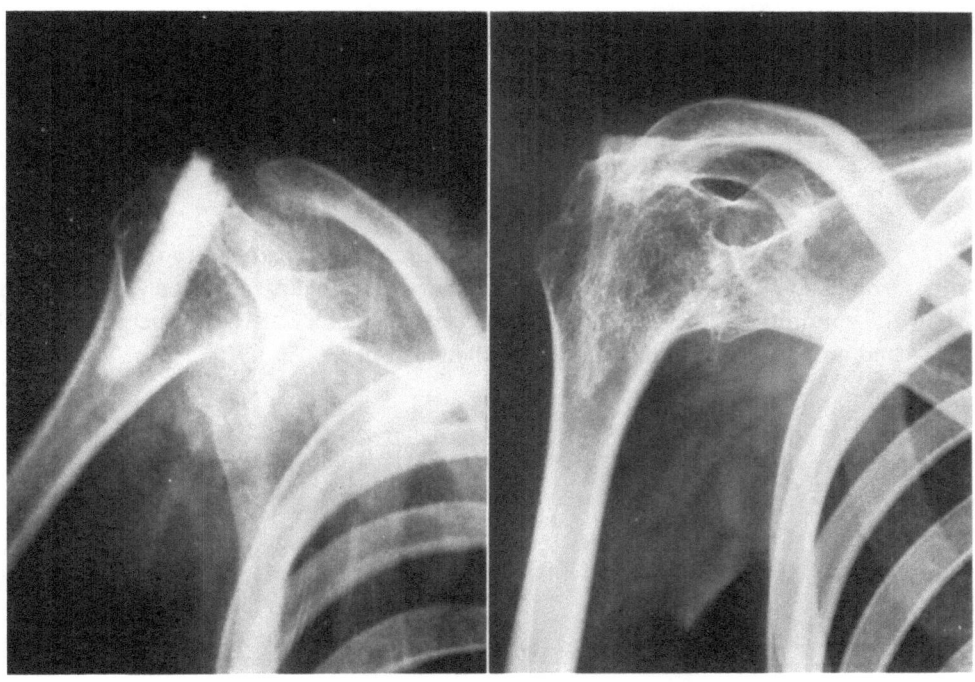

Figure V.15b

Figure V.15c

Diagnosis: tuberculous arthritis of the right elbow.

Previous history:

1956:   tubercolous arthritis of the right elbow, treated in a sanatorium.

Course:
2–5–1957:   admitted to Orth. Dept. W.G., tuberculous arthritis quiescent.
4–6–1957:   operation: resection of the right elbow joint, fixation with a homogenous graft, extending from the olecranon into the humeral shaft via the joint space. After-treatment in plaster and with abduction splint.
5–12–1957:   arthrodesis clinically sound.

Examination:
1–10–1959:   patient very satisfied, arthrodesis sound.

Radiographs:
8–5–1957:   figure V.16a, right elbow, joint destruction.
31–11–1957:   figure V.16b, graft in situ.
1–10–1959:   figure V.16c, bony ankylosis with continuity of bone tuberculae, graft still discernible.

Summary: Case of a successful intra-articular arthrodesis for a tuberculous arthritis of the elbow in a male aged 51.

Post-script: When we asked the patient to return for examination we received a letter from his wife stating that her husband had died of heart-failure on 2–2–1968, and that the condition of the arm had always been satisfactory after the operation and that he had been able to use the arm quite well in his work.

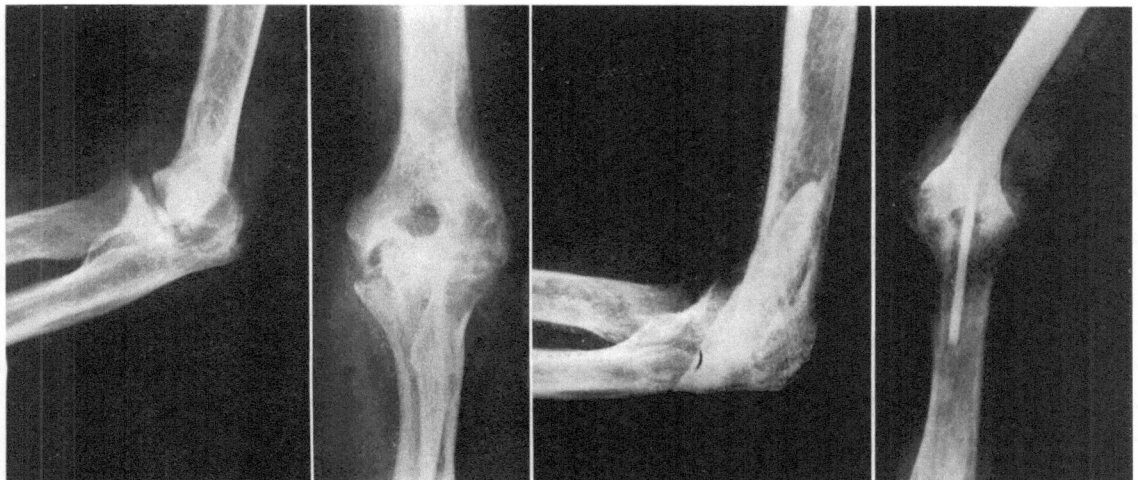

Figure V.16a   Figure V.16b

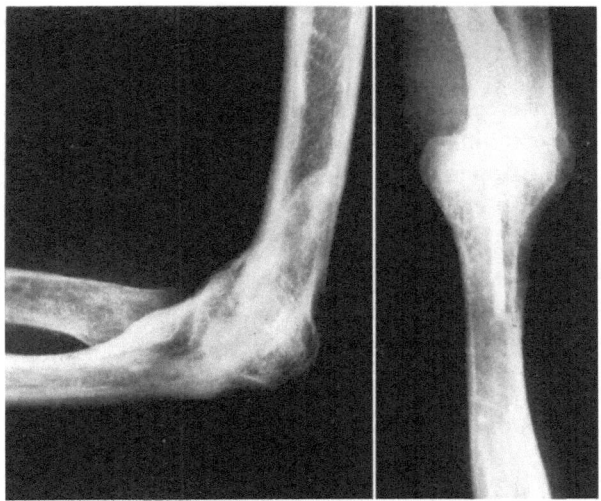

Figure V.16c

Diagnosis: tuberculosis of the right hip joint.

Previous history:

1944:   pulmonary tuberculosis.
1955:   tuberculosis of the right hip joint.
1956–1957:   treatment in a sanatorium.

Course:
26–7–1957:   admitted to Orth. Dept. W.G.; tuberculous arthritis in quiescent phase.
22–10–1957:   operation: extra-articular arthrodesis of the right hip joint by means of 2 homo-
              genous bone grafts extending from the major trochanter into the iliac bone, along-
              side the joint. After-treatment in plaster spica.
7–11–1968:   graft has acquired a functional form, there is now a definite bony ankylosis with
              continuity of the bone trabeculae.

Examination:
7–11–1968:   tuberculous affection looks healed, satisfactory arthrodesis.

Radiographs:
27–1–1956:   figure V.17a, tuberculous arthritis of hip in an active phase.
29–7–1957:   figure V.17b, right hip joint in a quiescent phase of arthritis.
22–10–1957:   figure V.17c, post-operative with grafts in situ.
22–9–1958:   figure V.17d, grafts assimilated, bony ankylosis.

Summary: Case of arthrodesis of the hip joint in a female aged 42 using 2 para-articular ap-
              plied homogenous bone grafts, which were well assimilated and adapted to a functional
              form; a very good result for a homogenous graft.

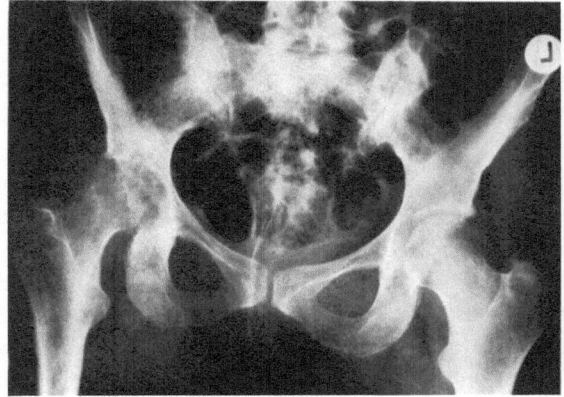

Figure V.17a

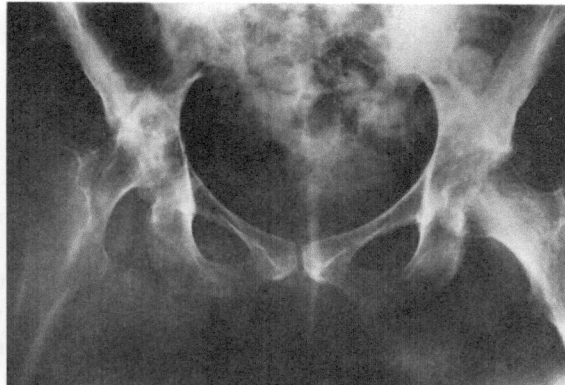

Figure V.17b

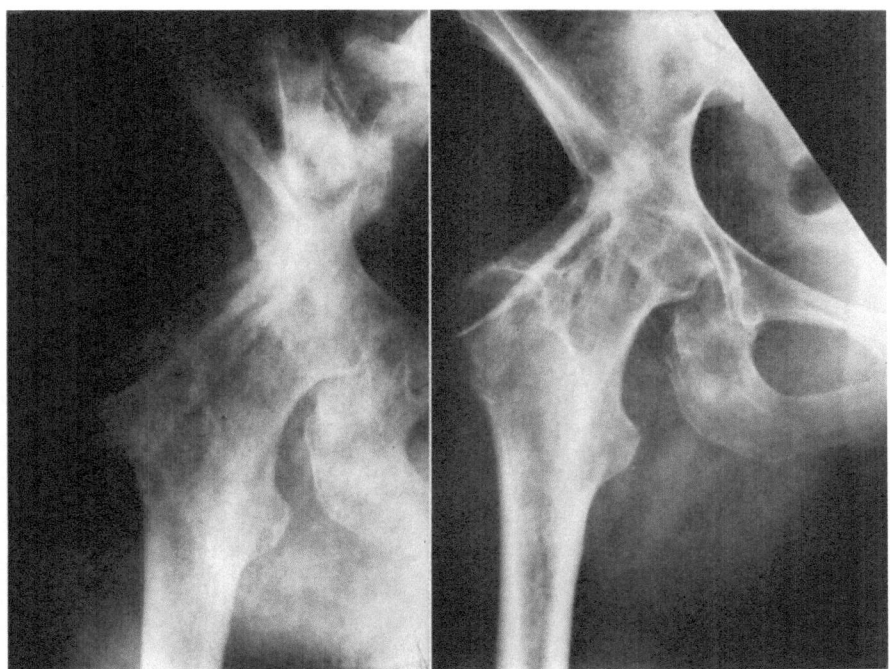

Figure V.17c   Figure V.17d

Diagnosis: dysplasia of left hip joint.

Course:
25–7–1957:   admitted to Boerhaave Clinic complaining about her left hip, osteo-arthritis caused by congenital dysplasia.
4–10–1957:   operation: arthrodesis of the left hip, exposure of the joint, dislocation of the femoral head, femoral head and acetabulum denuded of cartilage, reduction, fixation with 2 vitallium nails placed in a V-position with regard to one another, application of a homogenous bone graft between the major trochanter and iliac bone, plaster spica.
3–6–1958:   arthrodesis has succeeded.

Examination:
26–2–1969:   patient very satisfied, no more pain.

Radiographs:
25–7–1957:   figure V.18a, left hip, subluxation and osteo-arthritis.
24–1–1958:   figure V.18b, post-operative, two nails and one para-articular graft in situ.
26–2–1969:   figure V.18c, very satisfactory result of arthrodesis.

Summary: Very satisfactory result of *para-articular arthrodesis* with a bone graft combined with intra-articular mechanical arthrodesis. This was performed because of osteo-arthritis of the hip joint in a female aged 52.

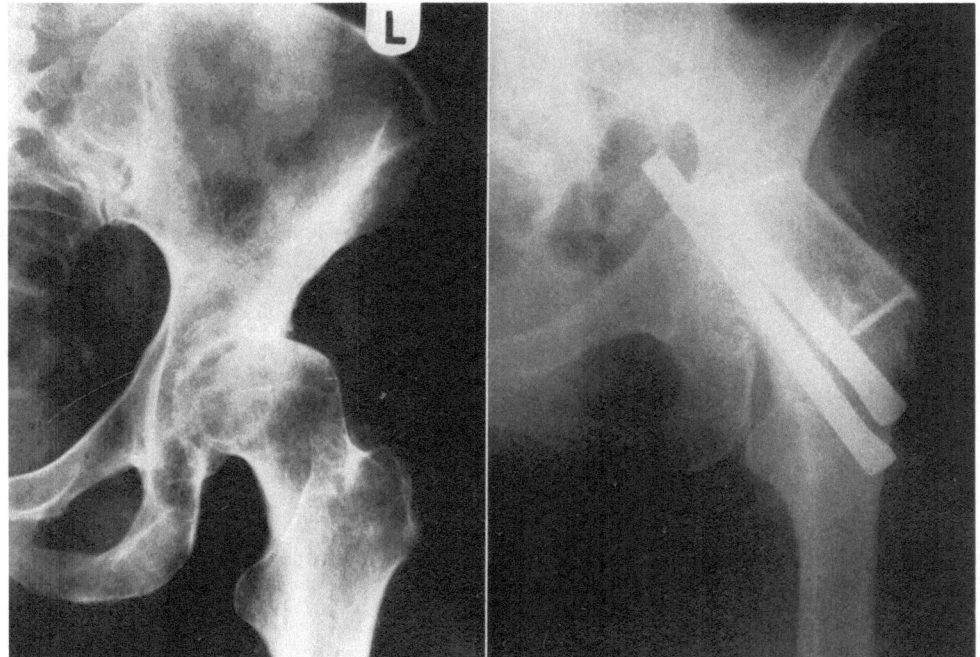

Figure V.18a   Figure V.18b

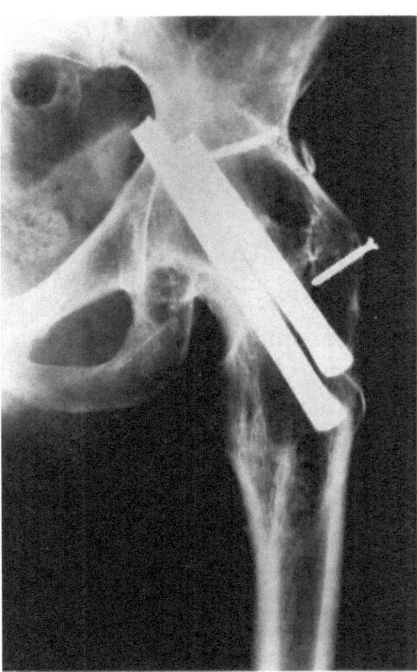

Figure V.18c

Diagnosis: paralytic scoliosis.

Previous history:

1956: poliomyelitis, followed by paralytic scoliosis. Indication for operation: progressive scoliosis and instability.

Course:

10–7–1962: operation: spinal fusion, 1st stage, D_1–D_7
2–10–1962: operation: spinal fusion, 2nd stage, D_7–L_1
30–10–1962: operation: spinal fusion, 3rd stage, L_1–L_4

Last examination:

14–3–1968: satisfactory spinal fusion with good correction and stability. Correction maintained, see table.

		D_2–D_{10}	D_{10}–L_3
8–9–1961:	before operation	140°	125°
14–9–1964:	2 years after operation	151°	136°
15–12–1966:	4 years after operation	151°	139°
19–3–1968:	6 years after operation	151°	136°

Light photographs:

13–2–1961: figure V.19a, before operation.
18–12–1964: figure V.19b, after operation.

Radiographs: Anterio-posterior photographs of the whole vertebral column with the patient in standing position.
8–8–1960: figure V.19c, scoliosis.
18–10–1962: figure V.19d, after 2nd operation in Milwaukee brace, graft in situ.
29–1–1964: figure V.19e, oblique radiograph shows successful spinal fusion.
14–9–1964: figure V.19f, same situation.
15–12–1966: figure V.19g, structural spinal fusion.

Summary: Case of application of homogenous grafts in extensive spinal fusion for a paralytic scoliosis, with very satisfactory result. A homogenous graft was inserted three times in succession, *from different donors*, without symptoms of intolerance.

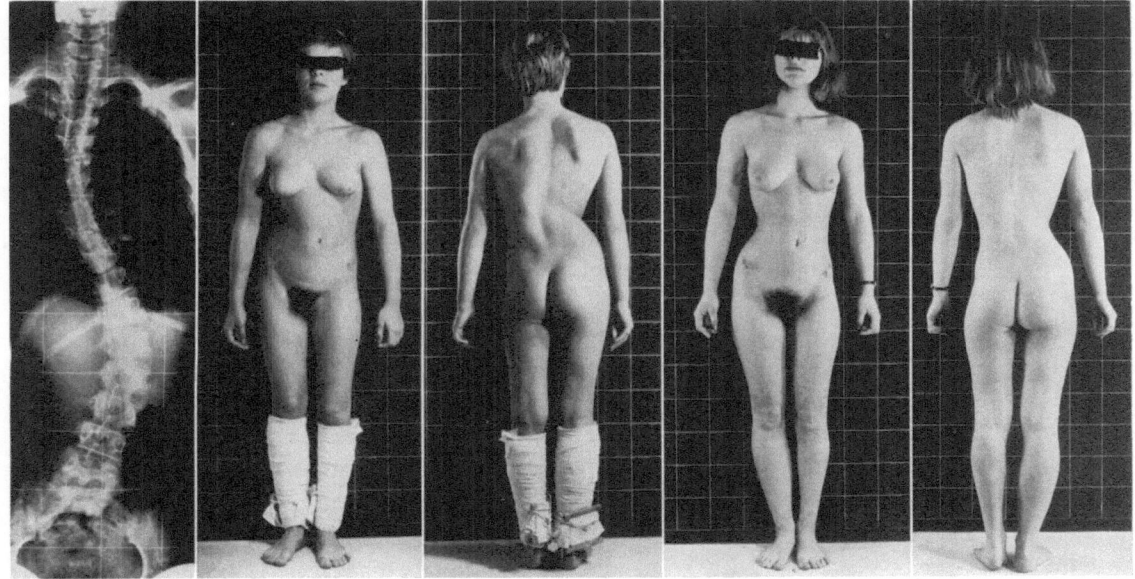

Figure V.19c   Figure V.19a   Figure V.19b

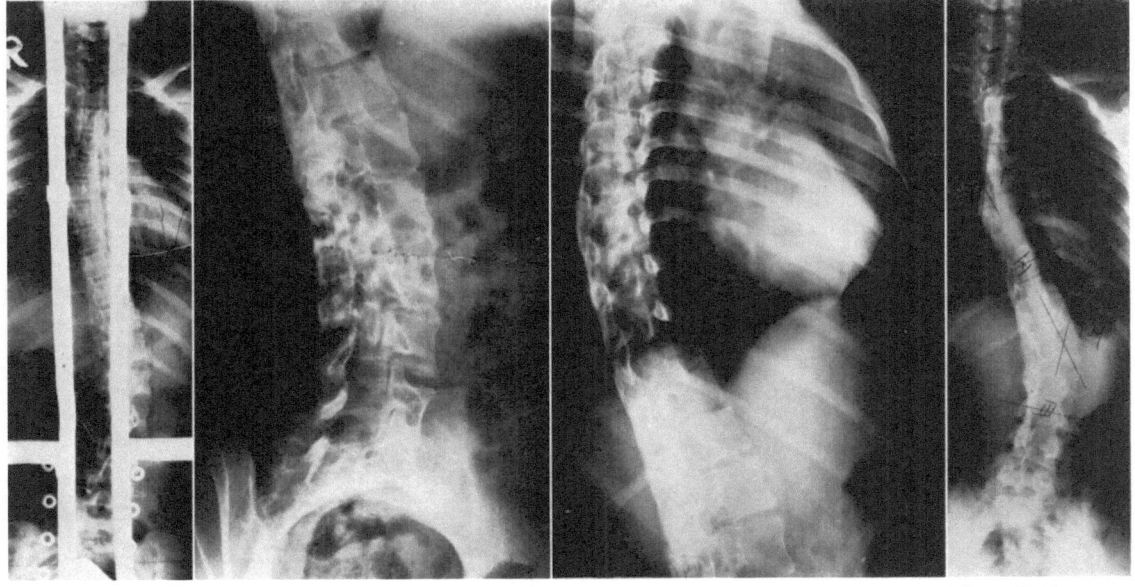

Figure V.19d   Figure V.19e   Figure V.19f   Figure V.19g

Diagnosis: paralytic scoliosis.

Previous history:

1957:   poliomyelitis, residual paresis of a great number of arm, leg and trunk muscles; prolonged rehabilitation has enabled this boy to stand and to walk again.

Course:

23–12–1961:   admitted to Orth. Dept. W.G., because of paralytic scoliosis, primary curve 135°, extending from D_5–L_4. Indication for spinal fusion: progression and instability.

23–8–1962:   operation: 1st stage, spinal fusion D_4–D_{10}, with homogenous graft.

9–10–1962:   operation: 2nd stage, spinal fusion D_{10}–L_4 with homogenous graft. Satisfactory course, stable spinal fusion achieved.

Examination:

8–11–1967:   patient well satisfied, vertebral column stable.

Light photography:

23–12–1961:   figure V.20a, before operation.

21–2–1964:   figure V.20b, after operation.

Radiographs:

6–4–1962:   figure V.20c, vertebral column before operation.

3–10–1963:   figure V.20d, vertebral column after operation.

24–9–1964:   figure V.20e, figure V.20f and figure V.20g, vertebral column, oblique radiographs show good consolidation of the spinal fusion.

8–11–1967:   figure V.20h, condition stationary.

Summary: Case of posterior spinal fusion in a patient with a paralytic scoliosis, which succeeded because of the application of bone-bank grafts; it would have been difficult to obtain sufficient autogenous material from this 'atrophic' boy.

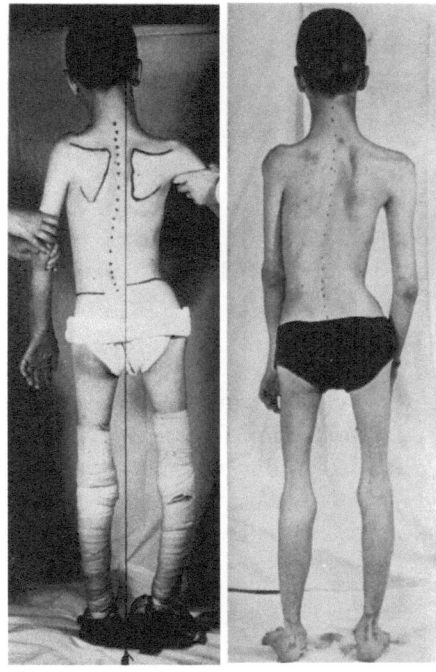

Figure V.20a   Figure V.20b

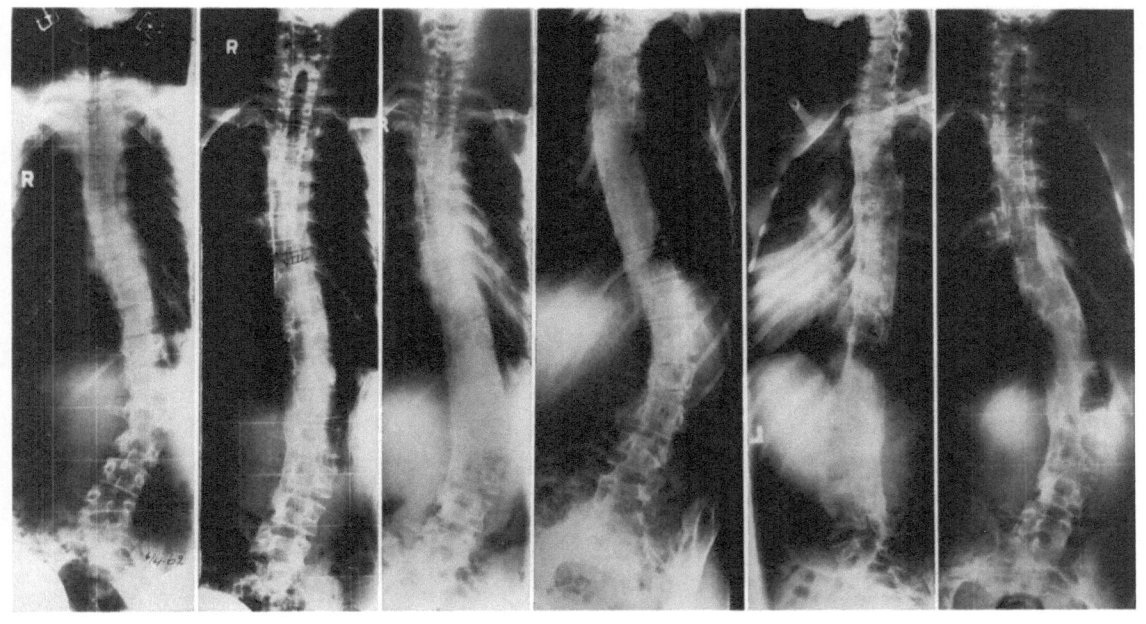

Figure V.20c   Figure V.20d   Figure V.20e   Figure V.20f   Figure V.20g   Figure V.20h

PATIENT V.21, BOY, BORN 21–8–1955

Diagnosis: paralytic scoliosis.

Previous history:

18–8–1956:   poliomyelitis, residual paresis of the abdominal muscles, muscles of the back and the right lower leg; scoliosis developed from a very young age, Milwaukee brace from November 1958

Course:

17–10–1963:   admitted to Orth. Dept. W.G. because of paralytic scoliosis. The primary curve 126° extended from D_6–L_1. Indication for spinal fusion: progressive scoliosis despite a Milwaukee brace, with desequilibration and an unstable back.

5–11–1963:   operation: 1st stage, spinal fusion from D_5–D_{12} with homogenous grafts.

12–12–1963:   operation: 2nd stage, spinal fusion from D_{12}–L_3 with homogenous grafts *from the same donor*.

Examination:

11–9–1968:   vertebral column stable, good correction achieved.

Light photography:

15–10–1956:   figure V.21a, paralytic scoliosis, pes equinovarus R.

8–3–1963:   figure V.21b, desequilibration, scoliosis, plaster-correction of pes equinovarus R.

28–10–1965:   figure V.21c, after spinal fusion, Milwaukee brace.

Continuation on page 92

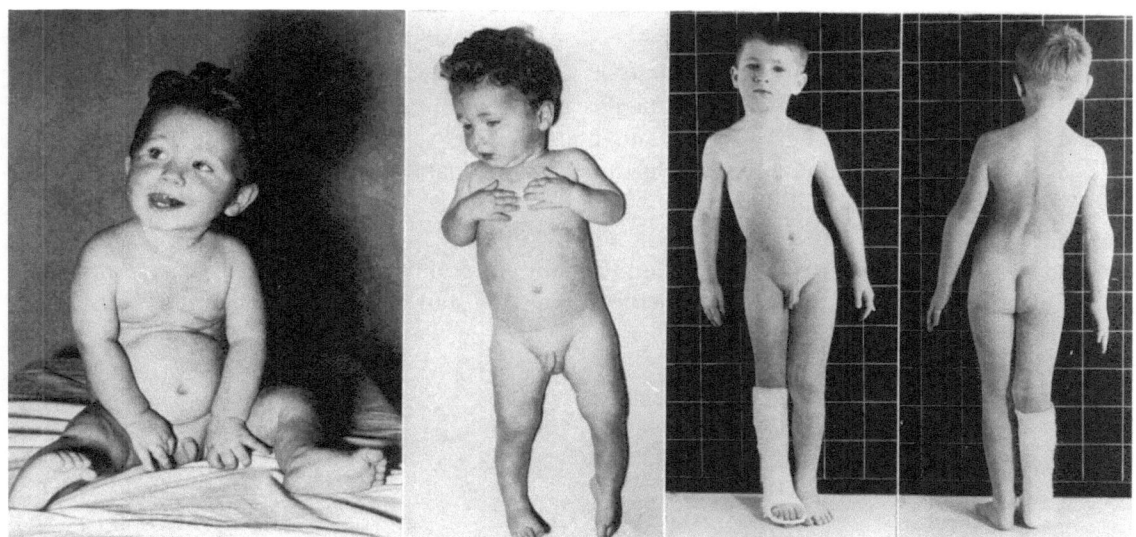

Figure V.21a   Figure V.21b

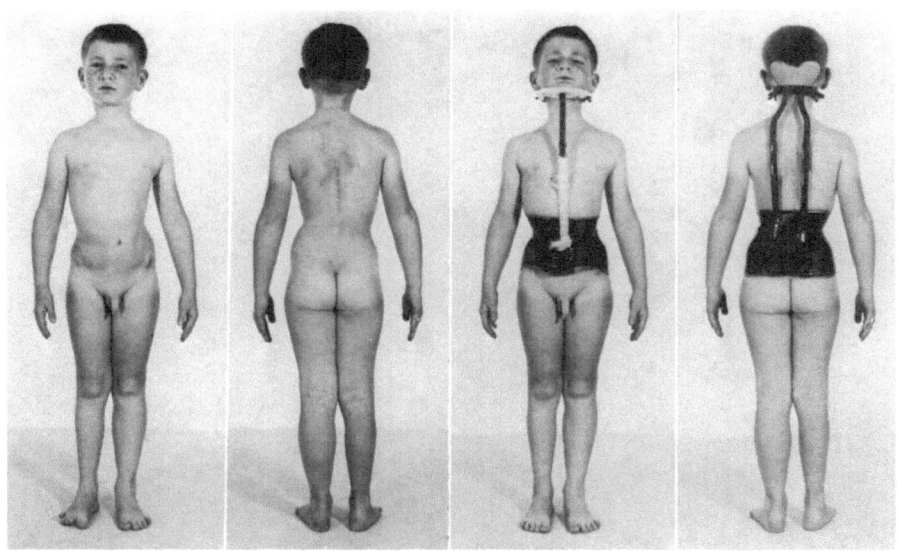

Figure V.21c

Radiographs:

30–9–1963:   figure V.21d, vertebral column, in anterior-posterior direction, standing, curve 126°.
23–12–1963:   figure V.21e, vertebral column, post-operative, in Milwaukee brace.
28–10–1965:   figure V.21f, figure V.21g and figure V.21h, vertebral column, anterior-posterior, standing, and oblique X-rays, satisfactory spinal fusion, primary curve 150°.
11–9–1968:   figure V.21i, consolidation.

Summary: Case of extensive spinal fusion for paralytic scoliosis in a boy aged 7, performed with homogenous grafts. Satisfactory correction and stabilization achieved, satisfactory assimilation of the grafts.

92

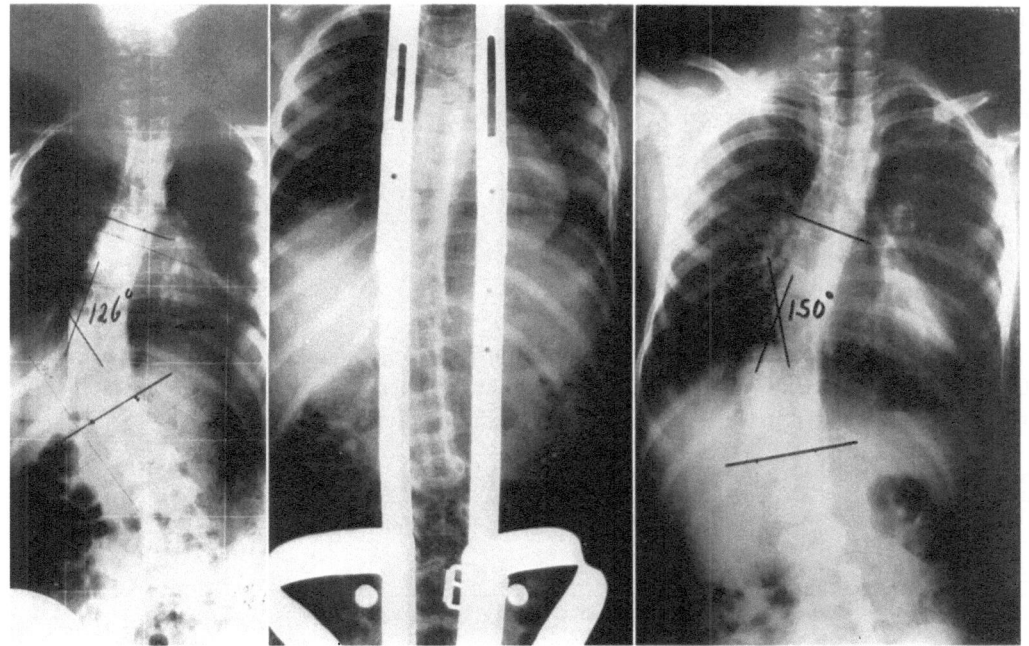

Figure V.21d   Figure V.21e   Figure V.21f

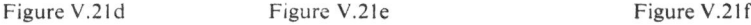

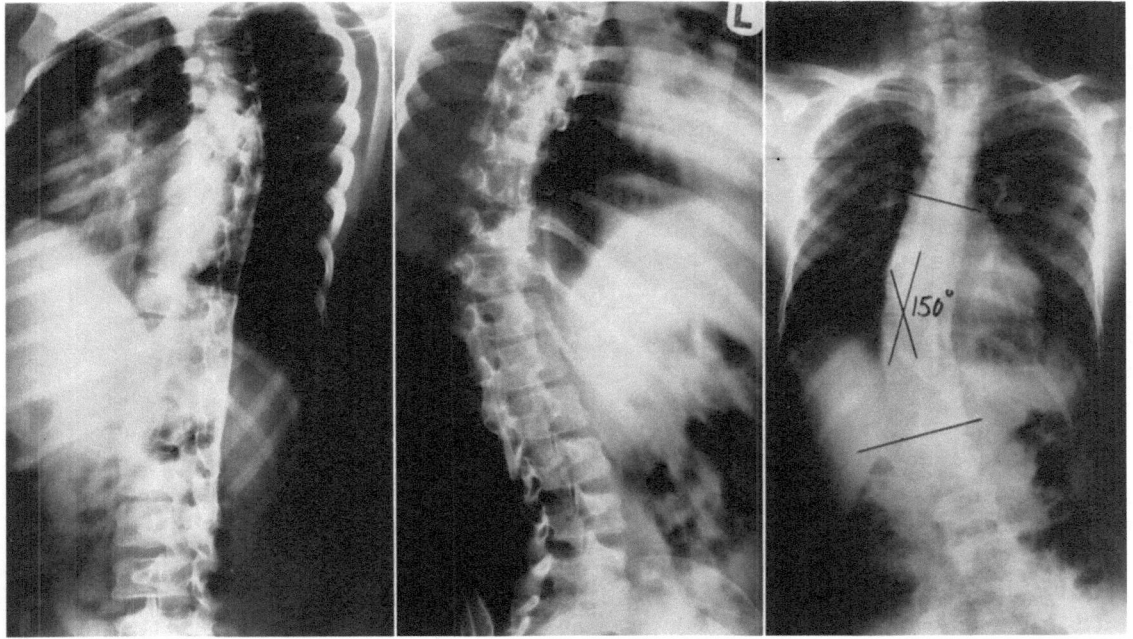

Figure V.21g   Figure V.21h   Figure V.21i

CHAPTER VI

BRIDGING A GAP IN THE SHAFT OF LONG BONES

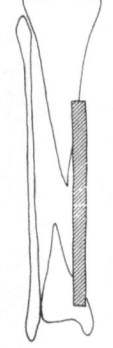

Scheme VI.1

This means the filling of a defect in the continuity of a long bone, either with autogenous bone from the patient, or with homogenous bone, the final aim being a transformation into a structural homogenity, with the graft serving as scaffolding-diagram (scheme VI.1).

Table VI.1. Statistics

	total	success	failure	unknown
autogenous	3	2	—	1
homogenous	3	1	2	—

Examples
Patient VI.1 and VI.2 bridging the defect with autogenous grafting.
Patient VI.3 to VI.6 bridging the defect with homogenous grafting.

CONCLUSION

Bridging a defect in the continuity of a long bone is such a major task, that nature must be presented with the best aids available, i.e. the solid mounting of autogenous bone. Even with autogenous bone the remodelling will be a laborious process over a long time with a fair chance of failure. Using homogenous bone nature will only be able to accomplish this heavy task in *the young child*. The osteogenic capacity of the young child enables it to build up the defect in the shaft into a normal tube of cortical bone with the aid of a homogenous graft. Related to this topic of bridging a defect are arthrorisis (e.g. posterior bone block for talipes equinus) and extra-articular arthrodesis.

Examples
Patient VI.7 up to and including VI.10, extra-articular arthrodesis.
Patient VI.11, arthrorisis.

The shelf operation in congenital dysplasia of the hip also belongs to this group. The operative procedure which is followed in the shelf operation is of importance, viz. the procedure represented in scheme VI.2, in which the acetabular roof is levered down and in which the defect is filled with transplanted bone, and the procedure represented in scheme VI.3, in which a bone graft is fixed into the pelvis proximal to the femoral head.
A third example is the arthrorisis of the ankle (patient VI.11). It is most interesting to compare the results of the autogenous and homogenous transplantations (Table III. 5, page 22). The percentage of success in the autogenous transplantations is 86.8%, in the homogenous transplantations 87.3%;

the fact that the percentage of success is greater in the homogenous transplantations as compared with the autogenous group attracts attention. Everyone with experience in this field knows that the result of a bone transplantation depends on many factors such as:

1. type of operation,
2. age of the patient,
3. type of graft.

ad 1. type of operation:
The condition of the wound bed in which the graft is embedded is particularly important; the fixation of the graft and undisturbed rest in the operation area also play a part; wound healing, the condition of the soft tissues, the vascularization of bone and soft tissues are factors which influence the result.
If we look further into the condition of the wound bed in which the graft is embedded, the operations using bone transplantation may be classified as follows:

a. graft completely surrounded by bone tissue.
b. graft along one of its long sides in contact with bone tissue.
c. graft at its extremities in contact with bone tissue.
d. graft at one of its extremities only in contact with bone tissue.

These operations, from a to d, present increasing difficulties for a successful outcome of the bone transplantation.

ad 2. age of the patient.
The younger the patient the greater is the possibility of a successful outcome of the transplantation. This means for the orthopaedic surgeon that he may successfully undertake transplantations in children which in adults are doomed to failure; this refers especially to group c, bridging defects.
The first type of operation is quite suited for the use of a homogenous graft, which is in good contact all around with bone of the host. The graft will unite with bone of the host and assimilate.
The second type of operation is less suited for a homogenous graft, a large part of the graft is surrounded by soft tissues, and it is probable that the projecting part of the graft will be absorbed. *Although we can show some very successful shelf operations in which bone-bank bone was used, we must admit that the results of the shelf operation using an autogenous graft are usually much more satisfactory.* Related to bridging defects is the extra-articular arthrodesis. In an adult, a homogenous graft will never induce such a beautiful remodelling as the graft has done in patient VI.10.

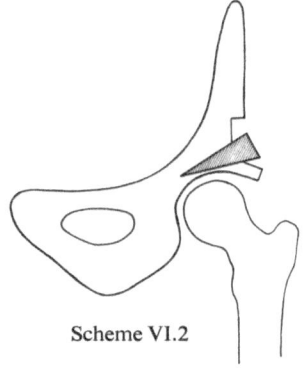

Scheme VI.2

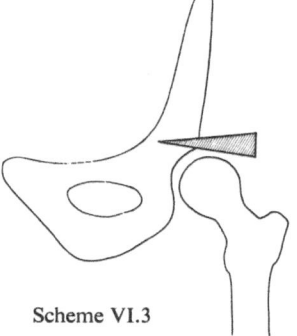

Scheme VI.3

Diagnosis: defect in the left femur.

Previous history:

7–2–1962:   accident, i.e. compound fracture of the left femur. A loose fragment of the femur was removed. From October 1962 under our care for reconstructive surgery.

26–10–1962:   operation: the defect was about 8 cm long, both femoral fragments were united by a bone graft as thick as a little finger, and the remaining defect filled with autogenous bone; graft and cancellous fragments were taken from the iliac crest. The post-operative course was satisfactory, after-treatment in balanced suspension with traction.

Examination:

12–12–1968:   good form and function of the left thigh.

Radiographs:

3–4–1962:   figure VI.1a, defect of the left femur.
9–11–1962:   figure VI.1b, post-operative.
28–10–1963:   figure VI.1c, bridging of the defect.
12–12–1968:   figure VI.1d, very satisfactory reconstruction of the femoral shaft.

Summary: Defect in the continuity of the left femur, operative bridging with autogenous bone, good reconstruction of the shaft *after 6 years*.

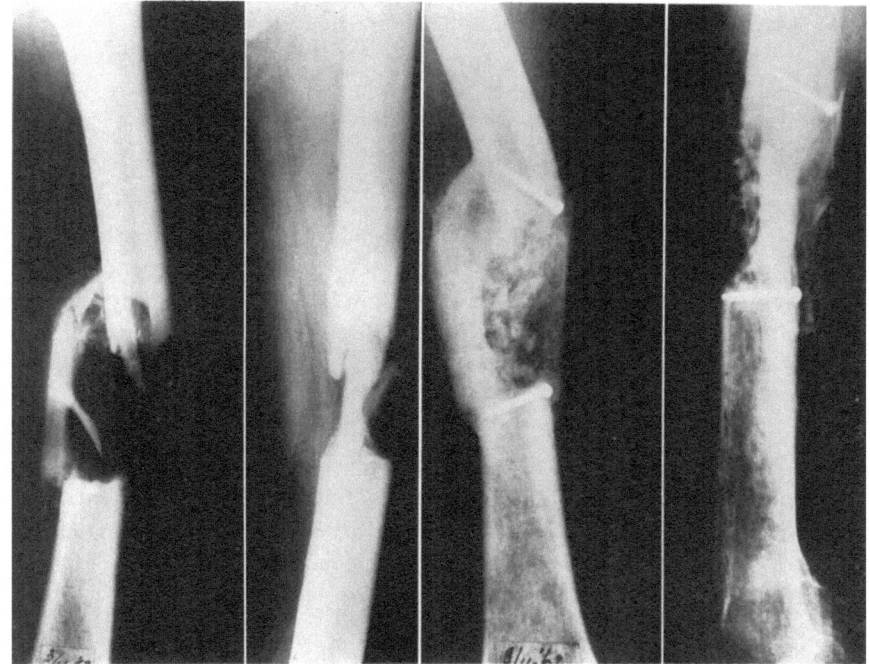

Figure VI.1a   Figure VI.1b

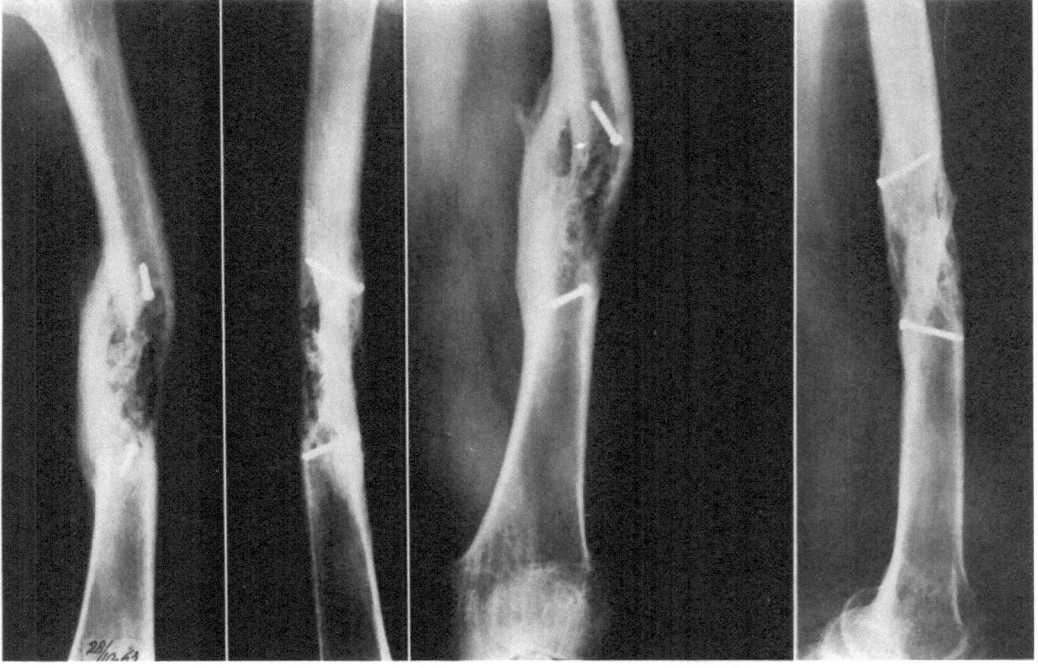

Figure VI.1c   Figure VI.1d

Diagnosis: fracture of the left lower leg with bone defect.

Previous history:

12–10–1963:   motor-cycle accident, with a compound fracture of the left lower leg with bone defect.
14–11–1963:   operation: osteosynthesis of the tibial fracture with an autogenous bone graft from the right tibia, there was a defect of 2–4 cm between the tibial fragments; this defect was filled with bone chips from the fractured fragments. After-treatment in plaster. Post-operative course satisfactory, primary healing. Fracture clinically united on 7–9–1964.

Radiographs:

18–10–1963:   figure VI.2a, fracture of the left tibia and fibula with loose fragments and a defect.
15–11–1963:   figure VI.2b, post-operative, graft alongside the tibia, bone chips in defect.
21–5–1964:   figure VI.2c, reconstruction progressing, not yet complete.
5–11–1965:   figure VI.2d, reconstruction completed.

Summary: Fracture of the left lower leg with a defect in the continuity of the tibia in a male aged 25. The defect was successfully bridged with autogenous bone. The reconstructive process required about 2 years.

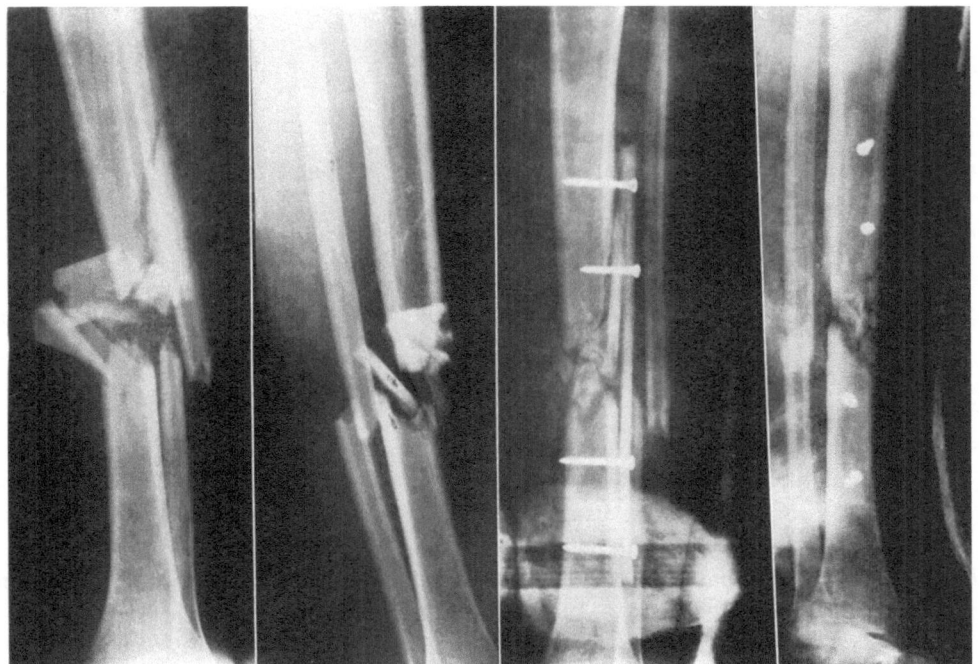

Figure VI.2a   Figure VI.2b

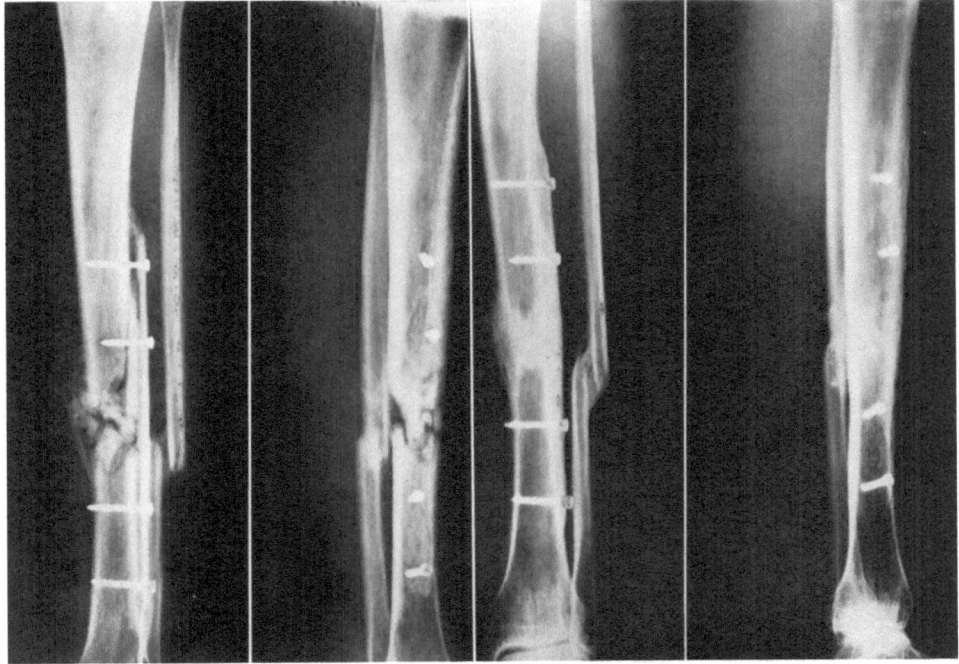

Figure VI.2c   Figure VI.2d

Diagnosis: pseudarthrosis of the right humerus with a large bone defect.

Previous history:

This girl had acute haematogenous osteomyelitis of the right humerus at the age of 6 months, the whole shaft of the humerus was destroyed. She came under our care in 1957 with the request that this large defect in the humerus should be restored.

Course:

15–7–1957:   operation: defect bridged with a homogenous graft; because the proximal and distal remnants of the humerus were very short, fixation could not be solid. Post-operative course satisfactory, the distal part of the graft took, but a pseudarthrosis developed at the proximal end with *epiphyseal growth*.

3–11–1958:   operation: repair of pseudarthrosis with bone graft from mother. Post-operative course satisfactory, graft takes. Humerus resumed growth.

Radiographs:

13–3–1957:   figure VI.3a, right humerus, defect-pseudarthrosis.

15–7–1957:   figure VI.3b, after first operation.

Continuation on pages 102-104.

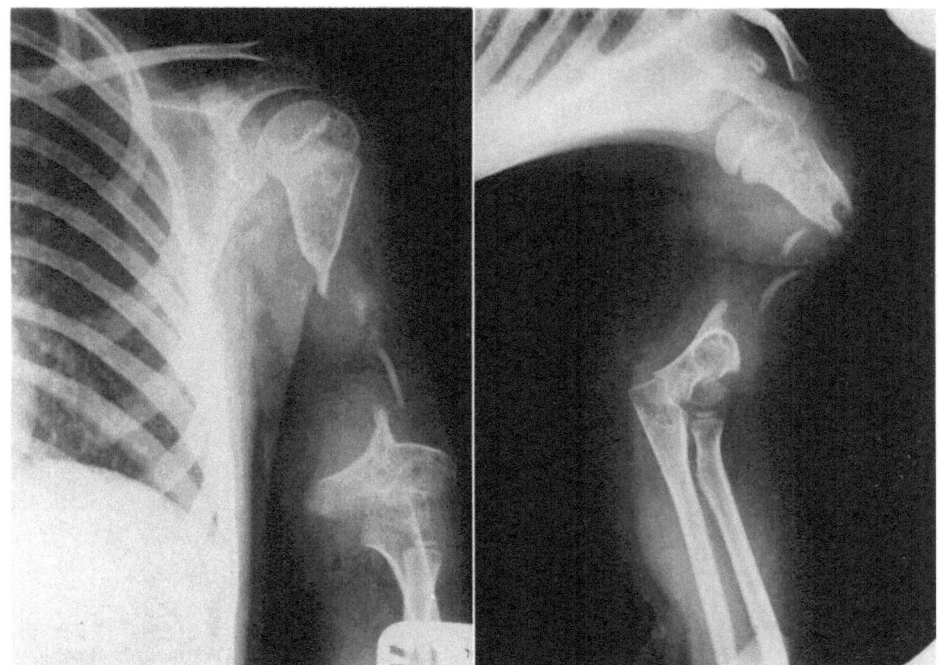

Figure VI.3a

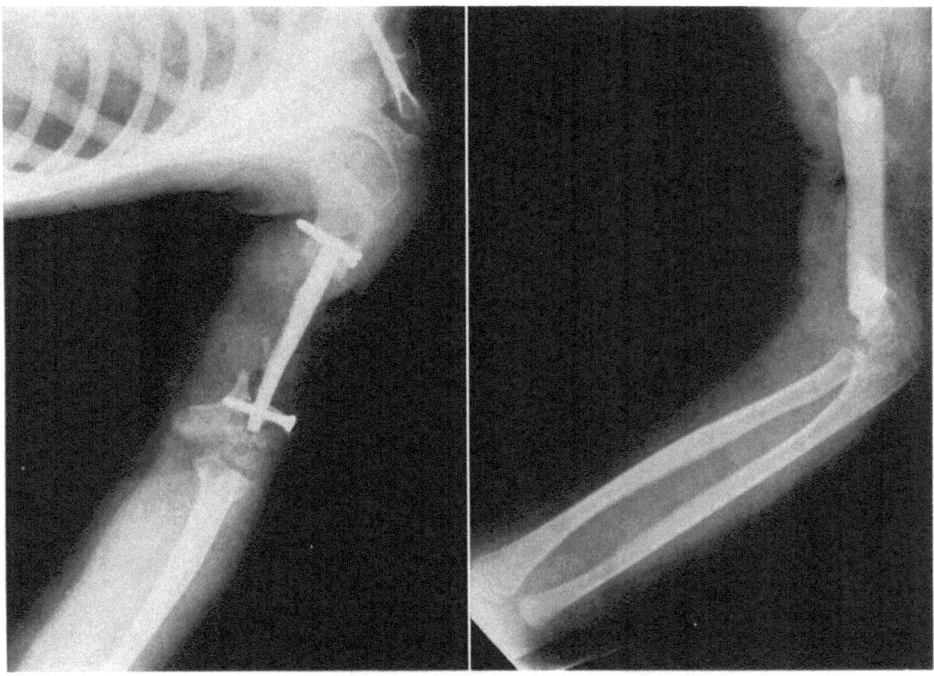

Figure VI.3b

101

15–7–1958:   figure VI.3c, graft has taken, merging with the distal humeral fragment, pseudarthrosis between graft and proximal fragment.
3–11–1958:   figure VI.3d, after second operation.

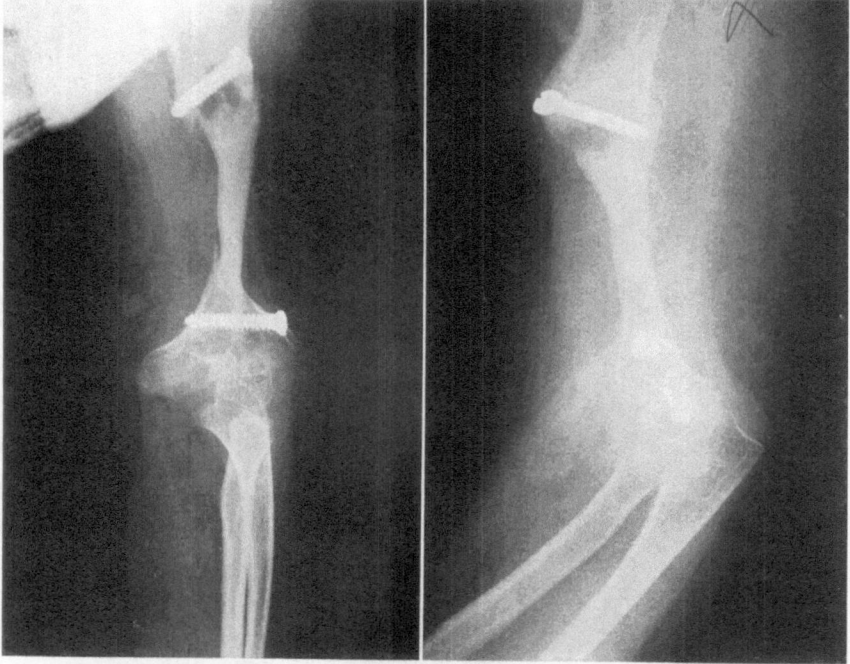

Figure VI.3c

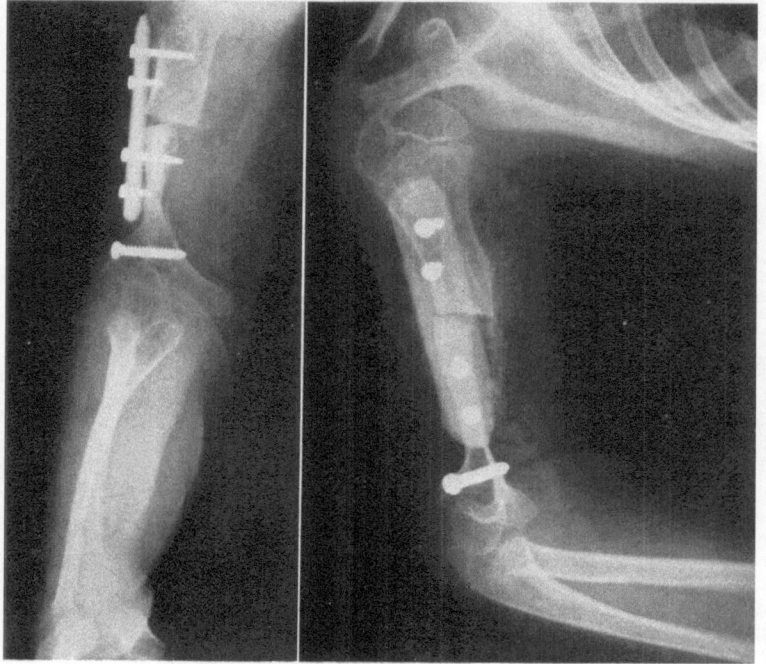

Figure VI.3d

17–6–1959: figure VI.3e, graft has taken, now consolidation proximally as well.

10–9–1962: figure VI.3f, a reasonable normal humerus has been reconstructed, graft no longer visible.

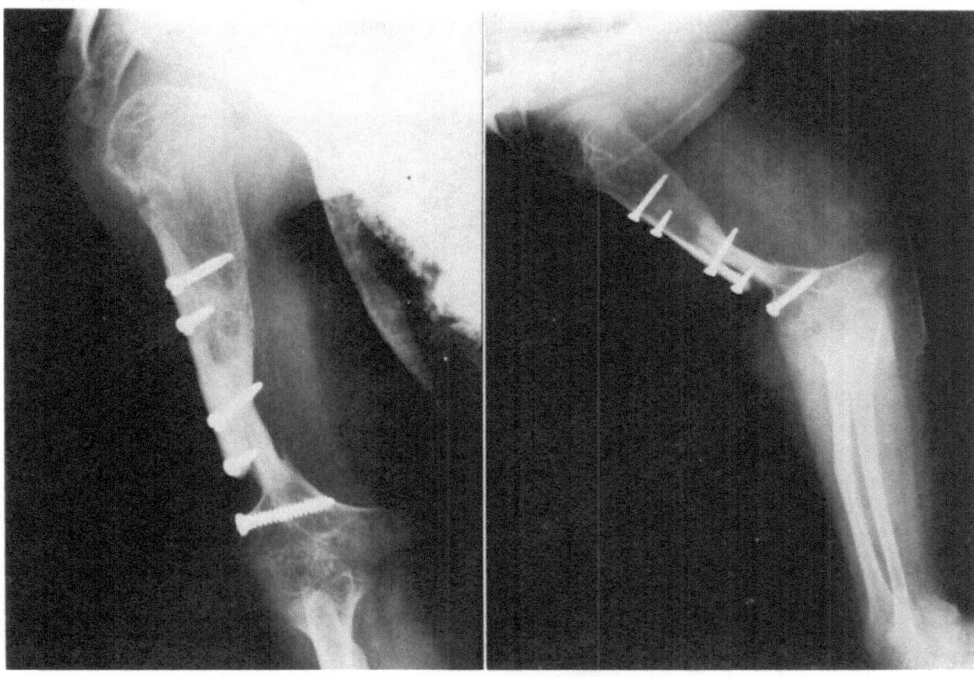

Figure VI.3e

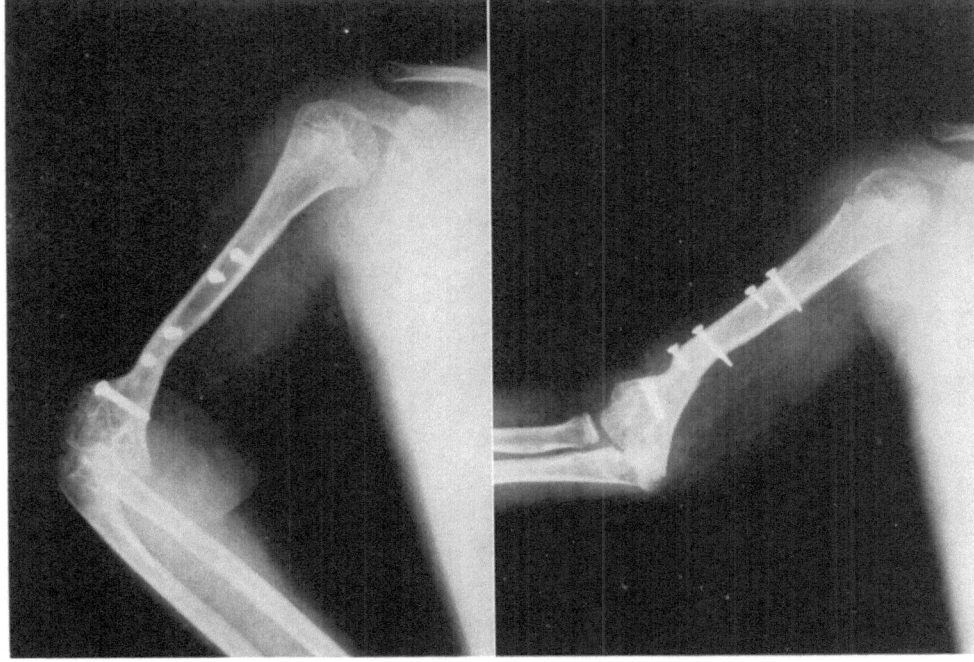

Figure VI.3f

28–3–1967:   figure VI.3g, satisfactory longitudinal growth of the humerus.

Summary: Defect in the continuity of the humerus in a girl aged 6. Successful homogenous transplantation despite a difficult condition, which succeeded because of the youth of the patient.

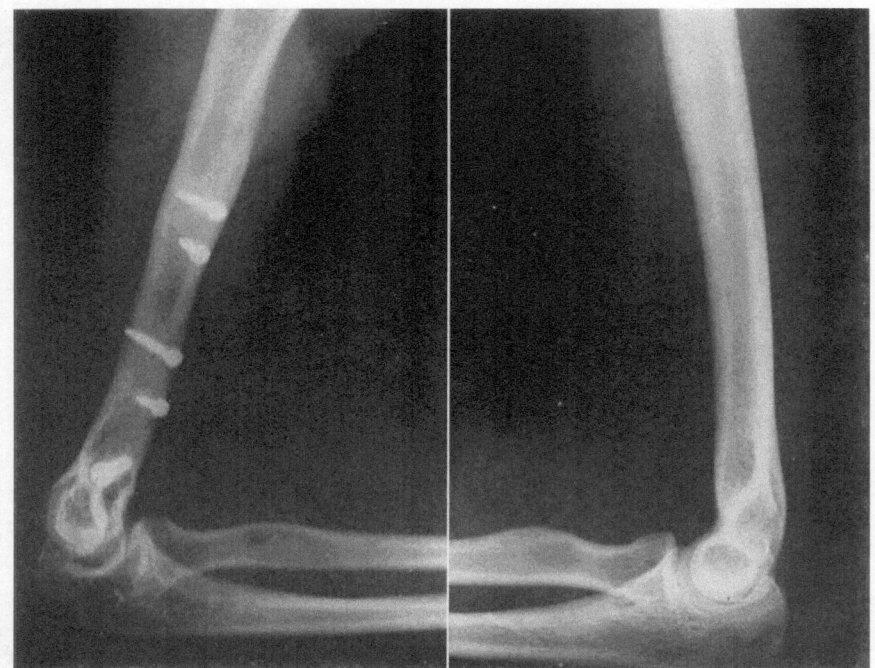

Figure VI.3g

Diagnosis: pseudarthrosis of right ulna with bone defect.

Previous history:

7–7–1955:   accident, fracture of right fore-arm, which resulted in pseudarthrosis which had been treated surgically elsewhere without success. Came under our care in 1958 for treatment of the pseudarthrosis.

11–7–1958:   operation: the bone defect in the right ulna 3 cm long, was bridged by a homogenous graft, and a block of cancellous homogenous bone was placed in the defect, after resection of the distal end of the ulna.

8–11–1960:   fracture of the graft at the level of the pseudarthrosis.

Radiographs:

10–12–1957:   figure VI.4a, pseudarthrosis of right ulna after failed bone-grafting.

11–7–1958:   figure VI.4b, situation after our operation, graft alongside the ulna with cancellous bone in the defect (bridging the defect).

14–7–1959:   figure VI.4c, graft appears to have taken; pseudarthrosis appears consolidated. However, no formation of a proper shaft with central cavity!

8–11–1960:   figure VI.4d, fracture in graft at level of the defect.

Summary: Pseudarthrosis of right ulna with bone defect in a male aged 31, bridged by cortical and cancellous homogenous bone. Failed. There was *no formation of a bony cylinder* with central cavity at level of the graft.

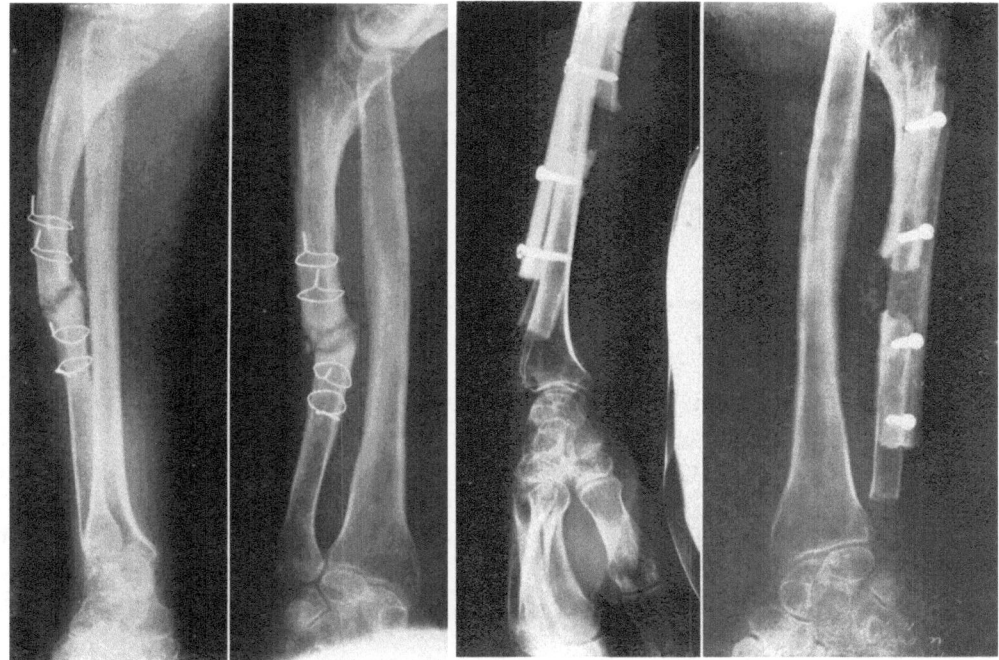

Figure VI.4a   Figure VI.4b

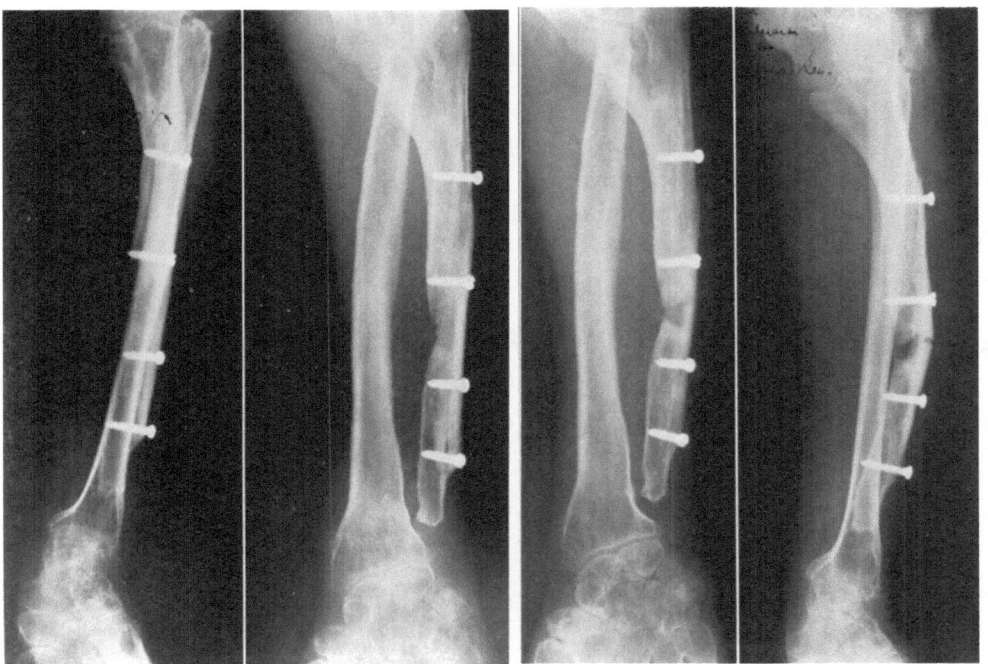

Figure VI.4c   Figure VI.4d

Diagnosis: fibrous dysplasia of left tibia.

Previous history:

Sept. 1958: swelling of left lower leg.
Jan. 1959: biopsy: fibrous dysplasia.
May 1959: excochleation (curettage) and filling of the cavity with autogenous bone chips.

Course:

29–1–1960: figure VI.5a, admitted to Orth. Dept. W.G. because of recurrence.
16–2–1960: figure VI.5b, operation: subperiosteal resection of 16 cm from the shaft of the left tibia. Reconstruction with 2 homogenous grafts and small fragments of autogenous bone from the iliac crest were placed as cross-beams in between. The remaining space was filled with homogenous cancellous chips. After-treatment in plaster. Fracture of both bone-bank grafts in 1961.
3–1–1962: operation: both proximally and distally to the defect, the tibia and fibula were joined with a fragment of autogenous bone from the right tibia.
Extension of osteolytic process in 1963.
2–8–1964: amputation because of recurrence of tumour.
The amputation specimen was investigated in the Pathological Laboratory W.G.: practically the whole tibia had been replaced by abnormal tissue, diagnosis: fibrous dysplasia.

Radiographs:

2–2–1960: figure VI.5a, process in shaft of left tibia.
16–2–1960: figure VI.5b, post-operative.
19–11–1961: figure VI.5c, both grafts fractured.
29–5–1962: figure VI.5d, post-operative.
10–12–1963: figure VI.5e, extension of osteolytic process.

Summary: Case in which bone grafting for bridging the defect failed in a male aged 47. The question arises whether the fibrous dysplasia together with the age of the patient should be considered the main reason for failure in this combined homogenous-autogenous grafting operation for bridging a defect.

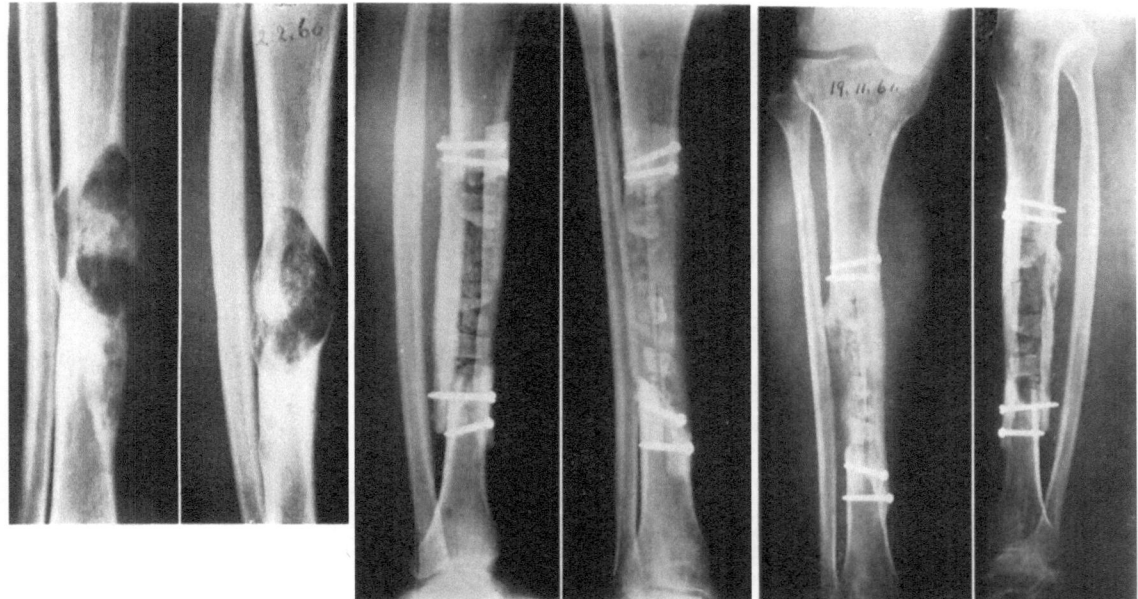

Figure VI.5a   Figure VI.5b   Figure VI.5c

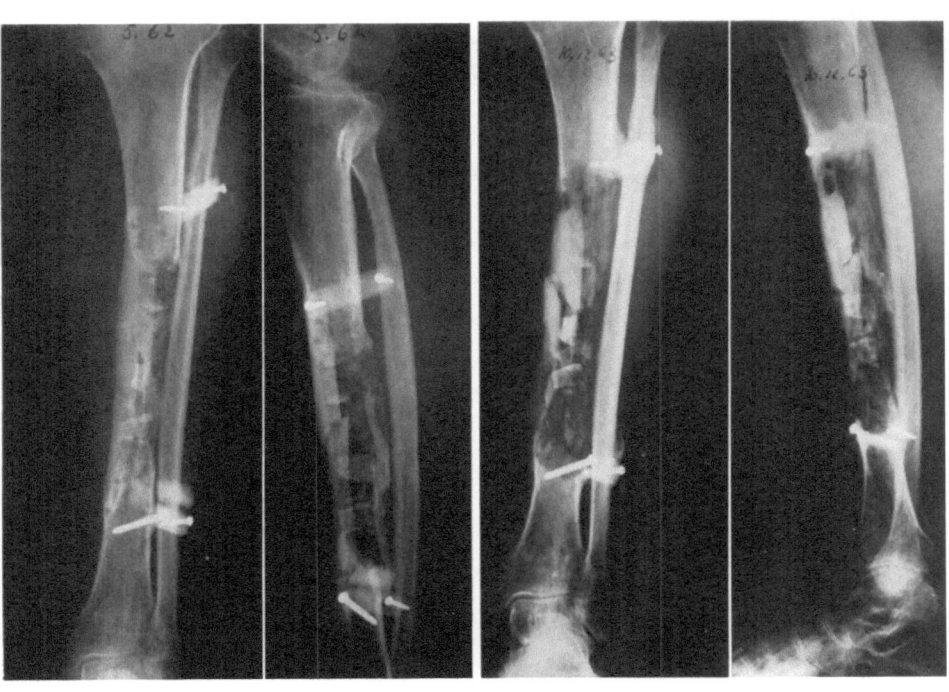

Figure VI.5d   Figure VI.5e

109

Diagnosis: congenital dysplasia of both hip joints.

Previous history: at the age of 2 it was found that the child had a dislocated left hip.

Treatment: reduction in general anaesthesia and plaster.

6–11–1946: shelf operation on the left side with 2 grafts from the patient's own tibia.

16–3–1951: the shelf had been absorbed, and a second shelf operation was carried out using a graft from the patient's own iliac crest.

Course:

3–11–1955: admitted to Orth. Dept. W.G. with bilateral subluxation of the hip, increased acetabular angle, previous operations failed because of resorption of the constructed shelf.

14–11–1955: shelf operation performed on the left hip with a graft of the patient's iliac crest.

4–10–1956: same operation performed on the right side.

Radiographs:

5–4–1954: figure VI.6a, bilateral subluxation of the hip.

14–1–1957: figure VI.6b, after shelf operation on left and right side, with autogenous grafts from iliac crest.

18–10–1966: figure VI.6c, last X-ray, with on both sides a good, functionally shaped shelf visible; the step on the left side has decreased; good functional remodelling.

Examination:

20–2–1967: subjective and functionally good result.

Summary: Case of shelf operation with autogenous graft, satisfactory result after 2 previous shelf operations (scheme VI. 3, page 95) had failed because of resorption. A homogenous graft would not have produced such a good shelf as has been obtained here.

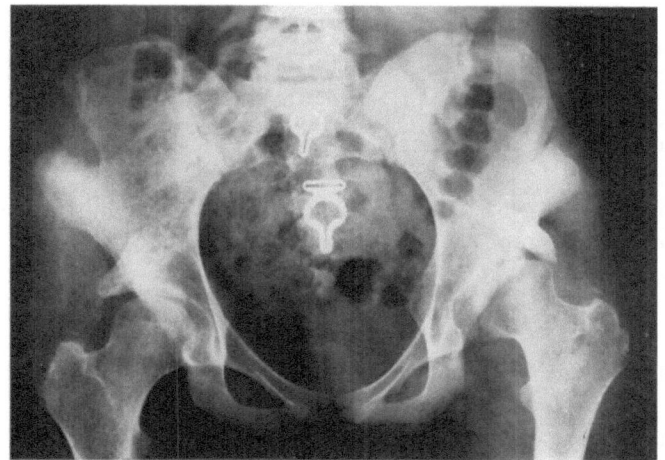

Figure VI.6a

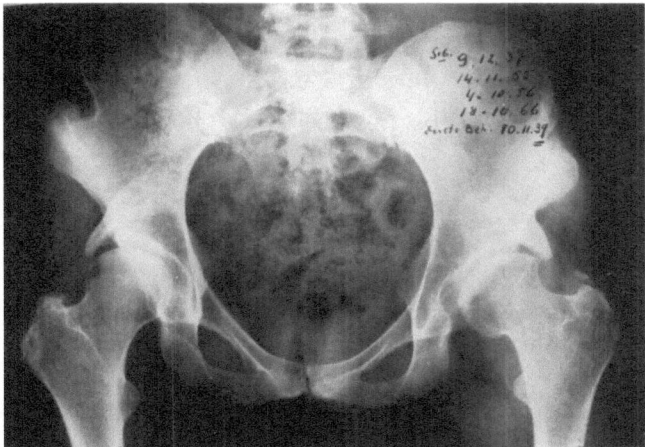

Figure VI.6b

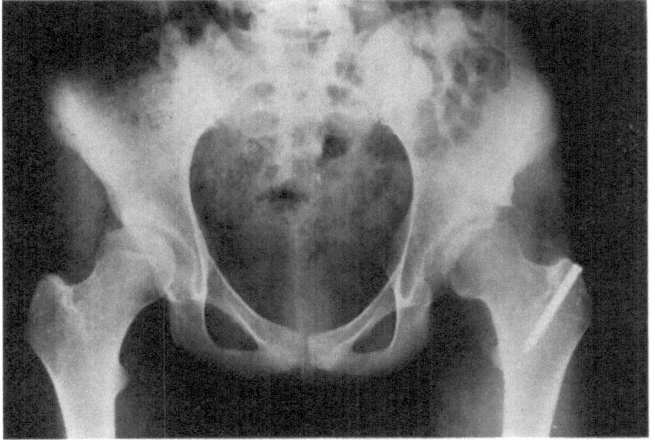

Figure VI.6c

111

Diagnosis: congenital dysplasia of the right hip joint.

Previous history: congenital dysplasia with dislocation of the right hip was discovered at the age of 17 months.

21–3–1950: reduction in general anaesthesia, plaster applied.

Course:

30–12–1953: admitted to Orth. Dept. W.G., subluxated right hip with pronounced anteversion, increased acetabular angle.

8–1–1954: operation: subtrochanteric osteotomy of the right hip, with varization and rotation.

28–9–1954: operation: shelf operation, with the aid of a chisel the acetabular roof (with markedly increased acetabular angle) was lowered, and the groove filled with small blocks of homogenous bone.

Examination:

9–12–1968: subjective and functionally a good result was obtained.

Radiographs:

8–1–1954: figure VI.7a, subluxated right hip.

7–9–1954: figure VI.7b, after varus osteotomy.

28–9–1954: figure VI.7c, after shelf operation, with autogenous and homogenous bone grafts.

6–12–1966: figure VI.7d, last X-ray, femoral head well centred in acetabulum, coxa vara, well-shaped acetabular roof, transplanted bone no longer visible.

Summary: Case of a successful shelf operation, procedure of *lowering the acetabular roof* and maintaining the shelf in position by bone-bank graft, as shown in scheme VI.2 (page 95).

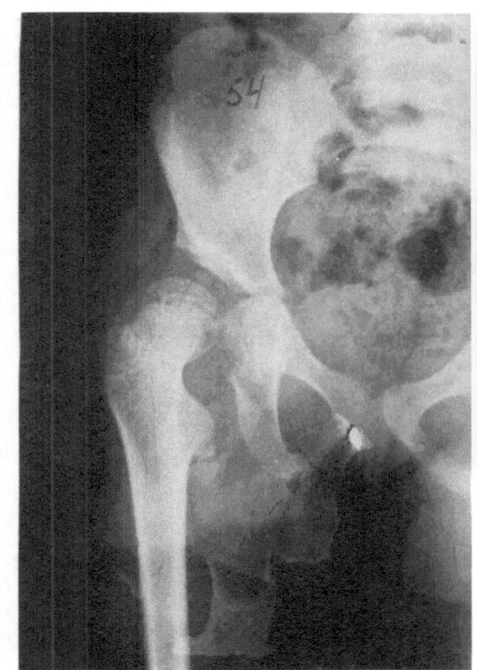

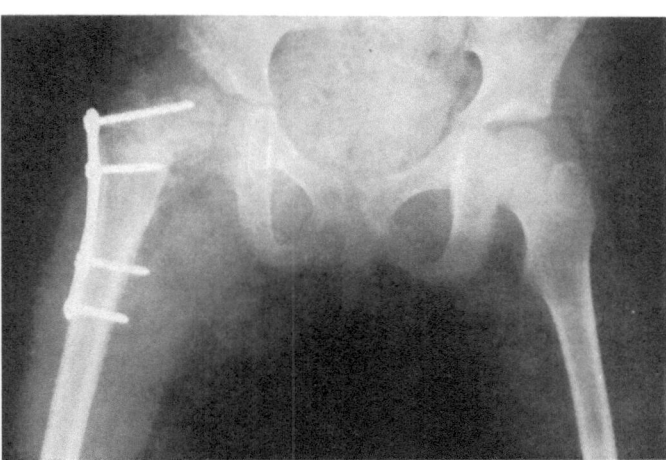

Figure VI.7a   Figure VI.7b

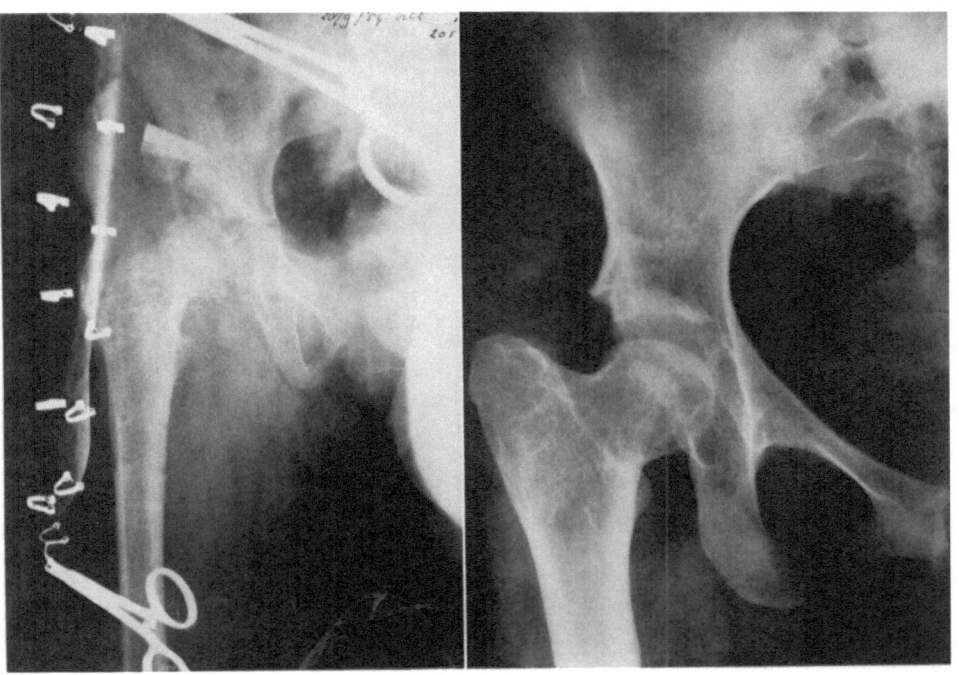

Figure VI.7c   Figure VI.7d

Diagnosis: subluxation of the right hip.

Course:

13–1–1960:	admitted to Orth. Dept. W.G., congenital dysplasia of the right hip with subluxation.
2–2–1960:	operation: subtrochanteric osteotomy with varization and rotation.
19–6–1960:	operation: the joint capsule and limbus were dissected from the anterior and lateral rim of the right acetabulum, and at the very edge of the acetabulum a slot was cut in the ilium, and a homogenous bone graft driven into this groove (technique as represented in scheme VI.3, page 95).

Radiographs:

21–1–1960:	figure VI.8a, subluxation of the right hip with coxa valga, increased anteversion, increased acetabular angle, poor structural development of the acetabular roof.
20–2–1960:	figure VI.8b, after osteotomy, femoral head now well centred in the acetabulum, still increased acetabular angle.
14–6–1960:	figure VI.8c, after shelf operation, large homogenous graft proximal to and quite near the joint.
13–10–1967:	figure VI.8d, satisfactory result, femoral head well centred, acetabular angle nearly horizontal, structural development of acetabular roof much improved, the shelf covers the head well, peripheral part of bone graft absorbed, varus position of neck and shaft decreased.

Examination:

13–10–1967:	a good subjective and functional result.
7–11–1968:	as in 1967.

Summary: Shelf operation using a homogenous graft in a girl aged 7, satisfactory result. A large part of the graft has been absorbed, but the functional part of the graft, however, (the part supporting the femoral head) is serving its purpose, and *suggests that it has had a biological action on the development of the acetabulum.*

114

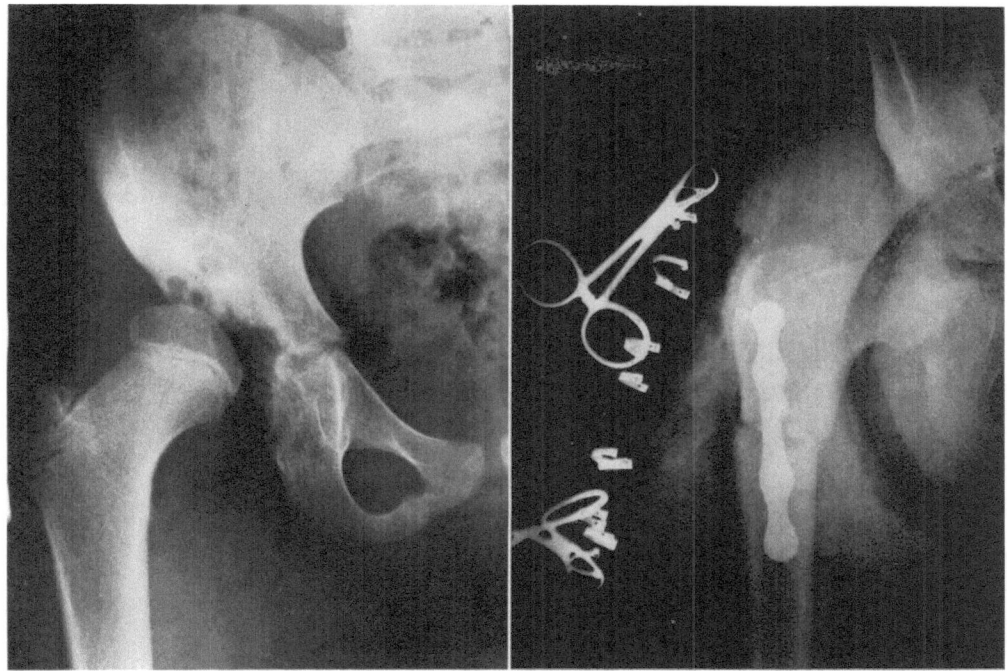

Figure VI.8a   Figure VI.8b

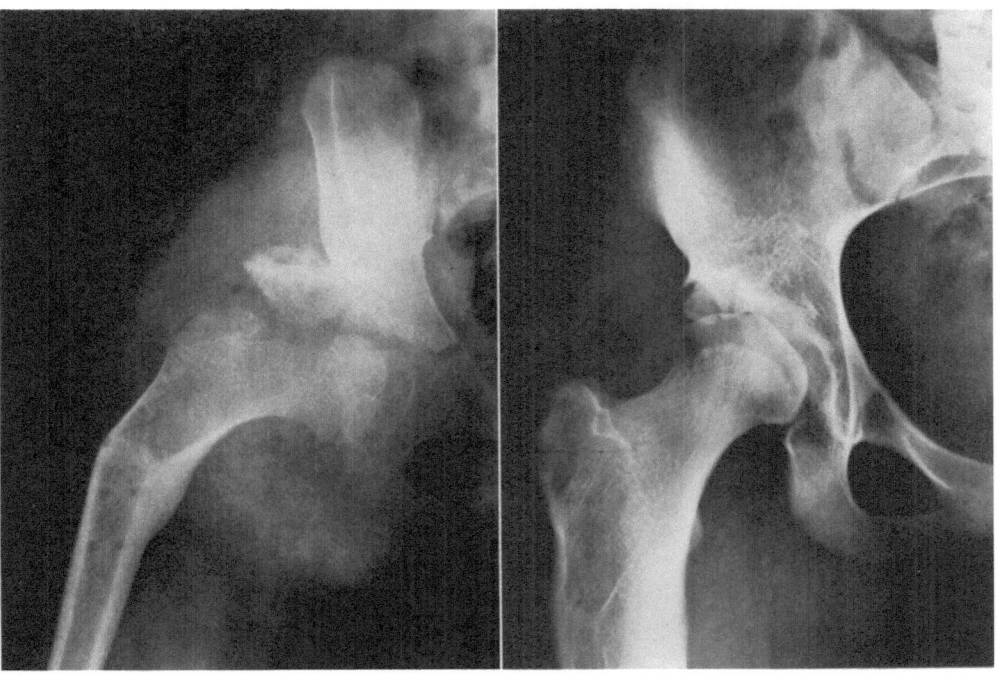

Figure VI.8c   Figure VI,8d

115

Diagnosis: subluxation of the left hip in cerebral palsy,

Previous history: a child with cerebral palsy, pronounced spasticity and grossly retarded motor development, who learnt to stand and walk at the age of 8.

Course:

20-6-1958:   admitted to Orth. Dept. W.G. with an adduction deformity of the left hip and imminent luxation of the left hip.

7-7-1958:   operation: tenotomy of part of the adductors of the left hip.

13-9-1960:   shelf operation on the left side, with bone-bank graft; close to the acetabular rim a slot was cut in the ilium and a bone graft inserted into this groove (technique as represented in scheme VI.3, page 95).

Radiographs:

5-9-1960:   figure VI.9a, subluxation of the left hip.

13-9-1960:   figure VI.9b, post-operative, homogenous graft well centred.

16-12-1965:   figure VI.9c, satisfactorily adapted shelf.

Summary: Case of a shelf operation with the aid of a homogenous graft in a child with cerebral palsy, which produced a good result.

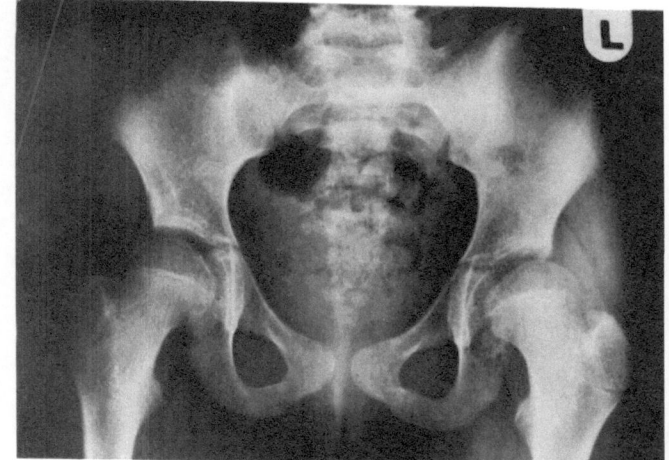

Figure VI.9a

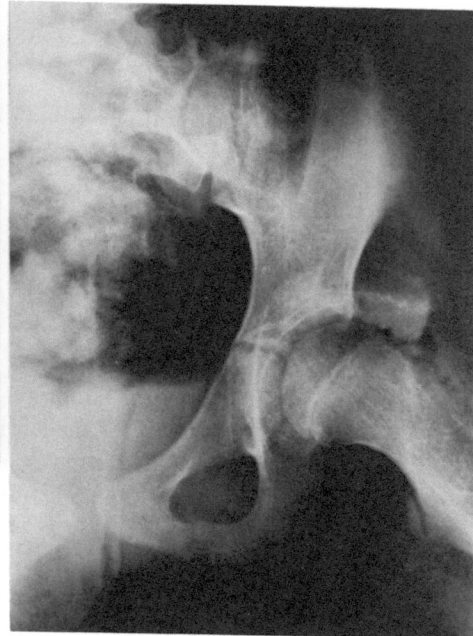

Figure VI.9b

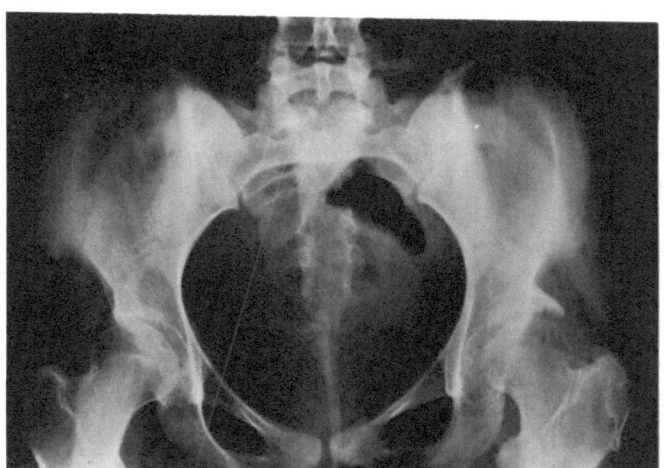

Figure VI.9c

Diagnosis: tuberculosis of the left hip joint.

Previous history:

1945:   pulmonary tuberculosis.
1947:   tuberculous spondylitis.
1951:   tuberculosis of the left hip, treated in a sanatorium.

Course:

29–5–1953:   admitted to Orth. Dept. W.G. with tuberculosis of the hip in a quiescent phase with fibrous ankylosis of the left hip.
3–6–1953:   operation: extra-articular arthrodesis 'Britain' with an *autogenous* graft from the tibia, after-treatment in a plaster spica.

Examination:

12–10–1961: quiescent. Stable arthrodesis.

Radiographs:

21–5–1953:   figure VI.10a, left hip joint after the tuberculous inflammation.
14–12–1953: figure VI.10b, post-operative, graft extending from femur to ischium.
12–10–1961: figure VI.10c, graft well assimilated, has obtained a functional form and has thickened, no bony ankylosis of the hip joint.

Summary: Case of a successful extra-articular arthrodesis 'Britain'. With an *autogenous* graft after tuberculous arthritis of the hip in a male aged 25. This hypertrophy would not have been obtained with a homogenous graft – we have here the formation of a 'functional column'.

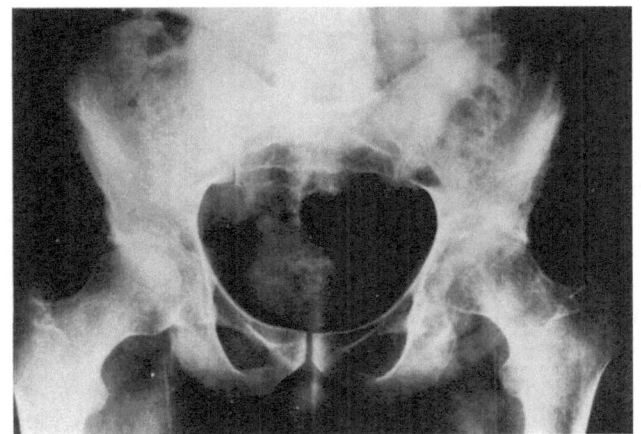

Figure VI.10a

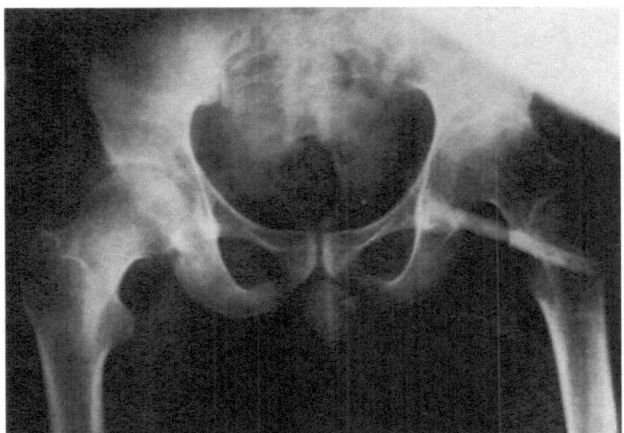

Figure VI.10b

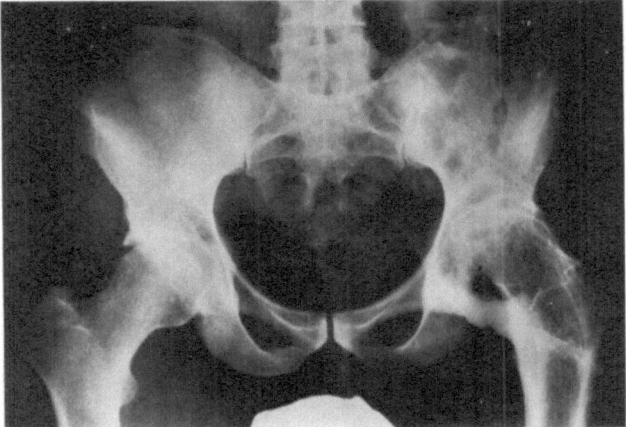

Figure VI.10c

119

Course:

Febr. 1959:   transverse myelitis.
21–6–1962:   pes equino-varus-paralytic and spastic.
9–6–1969:   8 months after arthrodesis with homogenous graft. Functional form.

Radiographs:

23–4–1968:   figure VI.11a, paralytic foot.
28–10–1968: figure VI.11b, arthrorisis after operation.
9–6–1969:   figure VI.11c, functional form after 8 months.

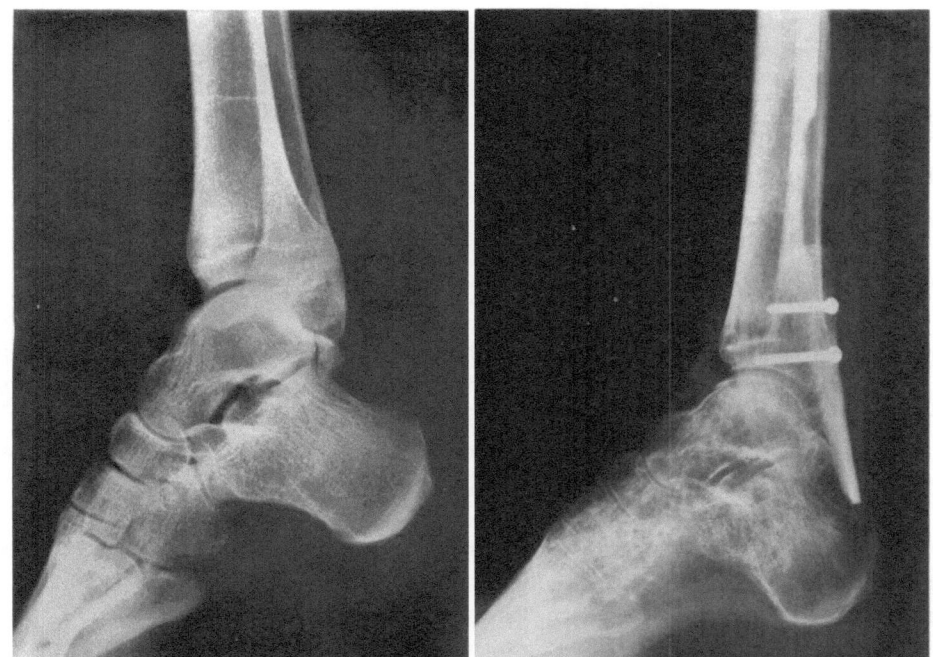

Figure VI.11a

Figure VI.11b

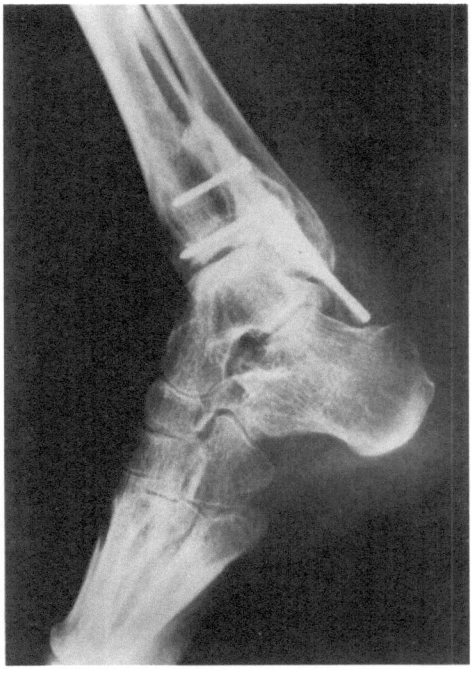

Figure VI.11c

CHAPTER VII

TISSUE CHANGES FOLLOWING
HOMOGENOUS BONE TRANSPLANTATIONS
HISTOLOGICAL AND MICRORADIOGRAPHICAL DATA

A. VAN DEN HOOFF AND R. STEENDIJK

From five patients who had received a homogenous bone graft, material for histological investigation was obtained during re-operation. The graft from one of these patients was also investigated by means of microradiography. The results of the microscopical investigation described below give indications regarding the tissue changes which occur after implantation of the graft and which in favourable circumstances result in merging of the graft with the bone of the host.

In the first patient (S. O.) spinal fusion with a homogenous bone-bank graft was performed at the age of 13 because of progressive idiopathic scoliosis.
The graft came from a male aged 16. Seven weeks after the first operation the second stage of the spinal fusion was performed and a biopsy taken from the graft. The histological specimen included the graft (sectioned transversely), part of the lamina and the spinous process and the soft tissues in between. The osteocyte lacunae of the graft did not contain living osteocytes. In the vicinity of the graft a multitude of new types of connective tissue had formed; immature granulation tissue of a fine fibrous texture, connective tissue of a coarse fibrous texture, fibrocartilage and also probably some woven bone, the latter in direct contact with the graft (figure VII.1). The new vascular connective tissue had in some places penetrated into the Haversian canals.

Patient 2 (P. van D.) was treated at the age of 16 for a fracture of the left humerus at the level of a solitary bone cyst. The cyst was opened up and emptied. A homogenous bone graft from a male donor aged 42 was inserted obliquely into the cyst and the part projecting outside the cyst was fixed to the outside of the humeral shaft. On re-operation, 2 years and 8 months later, the graft was found to be well assimilated; part of the graft was removed for histological investigation. Histologically that part of the graft was found to consist entirely of living bone. There were a few small, irregularly-shaped areas with large osteocytes and basophilic, non-lamellar intercellular substance: immature (woven) bone. By far the greater part of the bone examined consisted of normal Haversian systems arranged around bloodvessels, with normal osteocytes.

The third patient (A. T., patient no. 7, chapter V), was a man aged 87, who had fractured his right femur and who had an osteosynthesis performed with a homogenous graft. The donor was a man aged 47. Healing was satisfactory. One year and 9 months later he sustained a refracture of the right femur at the same level as a result of an accident. This made re-operation necessary during which the first graft was removed. There was a bony junction of the graft to the femur, the graft was white and did not contain bloodvessels. Microscopically the graft appeared to consist mainly of dead bone; the Haversian canals did not contain any blood vessels. Massive formation of young bone at the periphery of the graft was remarkable. This bone had the characteristics of woven bone: large osteocyte lacunae and interwoven fibrous texture; there were numerous bloodvessels, but lamellae could not be identified. Amidst this woven bone, remnants of dead lamellar bone were present (figure VII.2). At the junction of dead lamellar bone and living woven bone there was always a clear cementing line which – judged by the frequent appearance of ruptures – was not very firm. At the junction with the surrounding connective tissue all the characteristics of active formation of woven bone could be observed: the connective tissue was immature, with an abundance of bloodvessels and bone forming cells.

As the specimen did not contain the area adjoining the femur, no data could be obtained regarding the attachment of the graft to the femur.

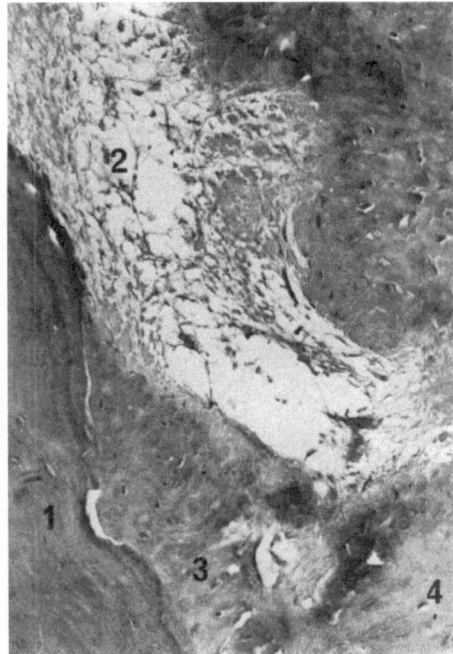

Figure VII.1. Patient 1 (S.O.). Reactions in the surrounding connective tissue, 9 weeks after implantation of a homogenous graft. 1: graft; 2: immature connective tissue; 3: woven bone; 4: cartilage. 120 ×.

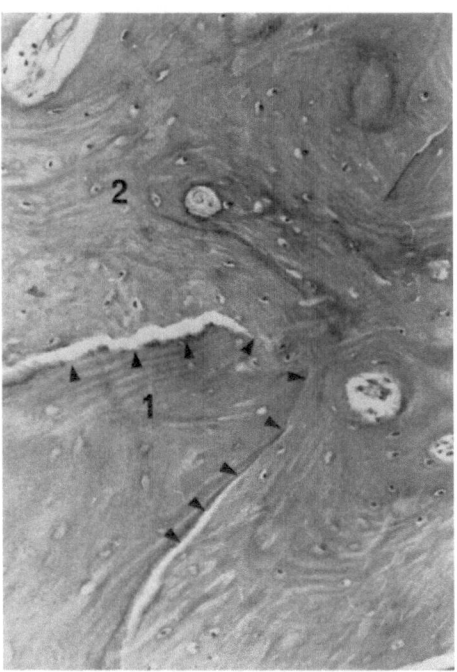

Figure VII.2. Patient 3 (A.T., no. 7, chapter V). Material from a homogenous graft after 21 months. 1: original material from graft; 2: penetration of woven bone. 120 ×.

From the fourth patient (M. M., patient no. 6, chapter V) material was available for histological as well as microradiographical examination. This patient was aged 18 and had sustained a fracture of the left femur which was treated by osteosynthesis using a homogenous bone graft obtained from a 41-year-oldman. $3\frac{1}{2}$ years later, after a refracture following minor trauma, the graft was removed and the whole of it became available for microscopical examination.

Macroscopically the graft appeared completely reconstructed at its extremities and well merged with the underlying femur. At the level of the fracture the graft was dead and had not merged. Microscopically it was not possible to see obvious differences between the extremities and the central part of the graft. All sections showed lamellar bone that was mainly dead. Locally there were large irregularly shaped cavities filled with vascular connective tissue in which many osteoclasts were present. In other areas bone apposition by osteoblasts was seen in these resorption lacunae. Furthermore there were small areas of living bone, which had been deposited concentrically around bloodvessels within the dead bone, from which it was separated by irregular cementing lines. There were also small centres of concentric active bone apposition around bloodvessels.

This patient's microradiographic data are particularly interesting. Transverse sections were made at various levels of the graft. In several areas on the outer surface of the graft woven bone had been formed (fig. VII.3). It was clearly visible in places that this woven bone was growing into the graft via canals which were present in the graft.

In the central canals of quite a number of the original osteones of the graft, amorphous calcium compounds of a high density had been deposited (fig. VII.4). Elsewhere, generally at the surface of the graft, there were large resorption cavities of an irregular shape (fig. VII.5). Within many of these resorption cavities formation of new bone had taken place, which at the periphery often showed the characteristics of woven bone, but more centrally appeared to be lamellar bone. In between these cavities and the areas of formation of new bone, the original tissue of the graft was still present. Particularly interesting were the histological specimens of the fifth patient (B.H.S., patient no. 12, chapter V), a man aged 41, who had a pseudarthrosis of the left humerus which was treated with a

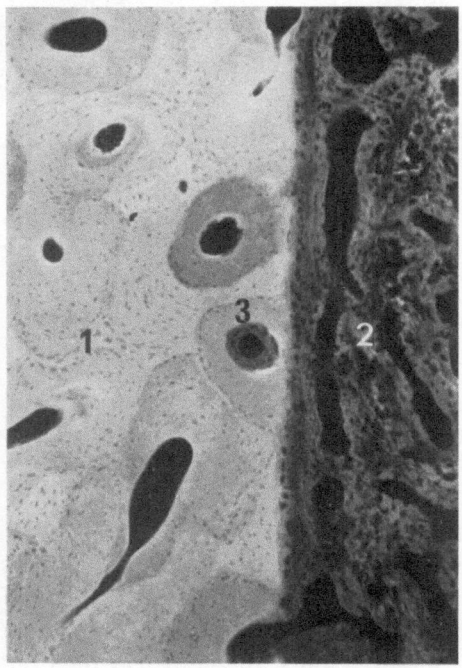

F gure VII.3. Patient 4 (M.M., no. 6, chapter V). Microradiograph. 1: homogenous graft; 2: woven bone (lower density of calcium, large osteocyte lacunae); 3: penetration of woven bone into the Haversian canals of the graft. 60 ×.

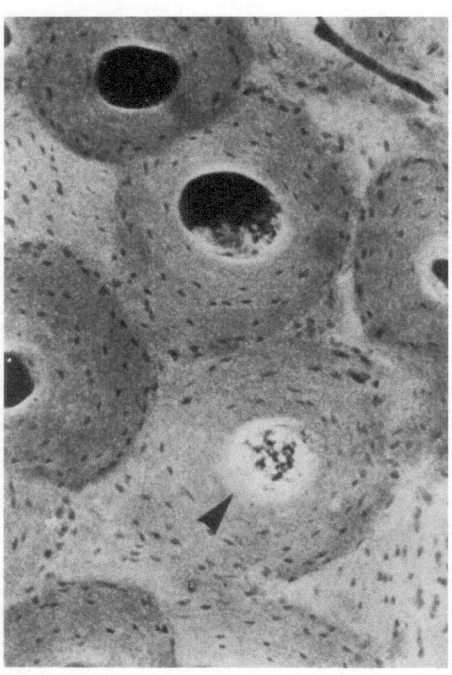

Figure VII.4. Patient 4 (M.M., no. 6, chapter V). Microradiograph. Dense calcified deposits in Haversian canal of graft (arrow). 120 ×.

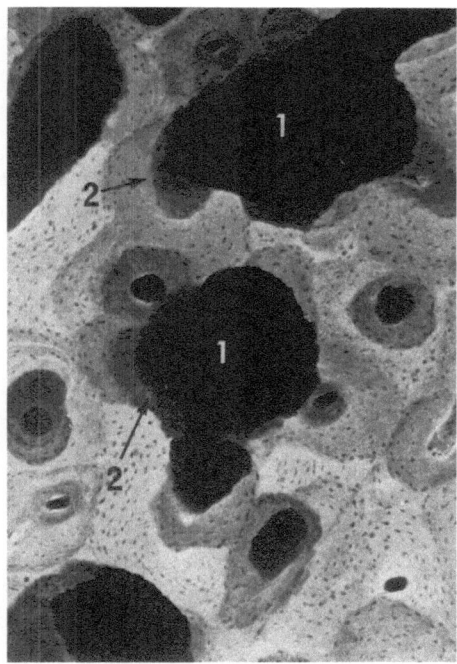

Figure VII.5. Patient 4 (M.M., no. 6, chapter V). Microradiograph. 1: resorption cavities in the graft; 2: local apposition of new bone. 60 ×.

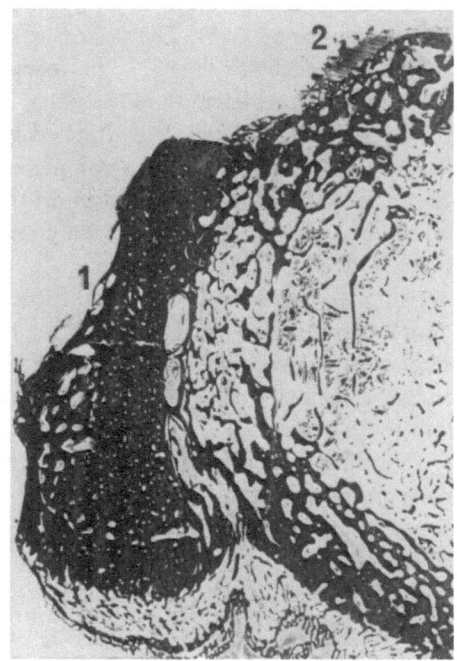

Figure VII.6. Patient 5 (B.H.S., no. 12, chapter V). Survey picture. The homogenous graft (1) is completely united with the humerus (2). Near this union the humerus is porotic. 4 ×.

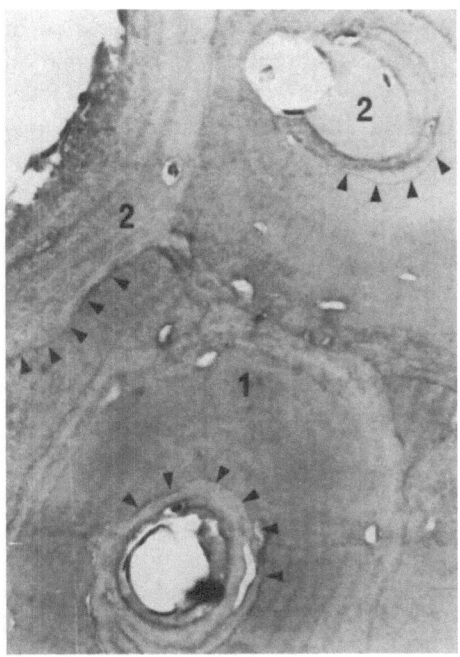

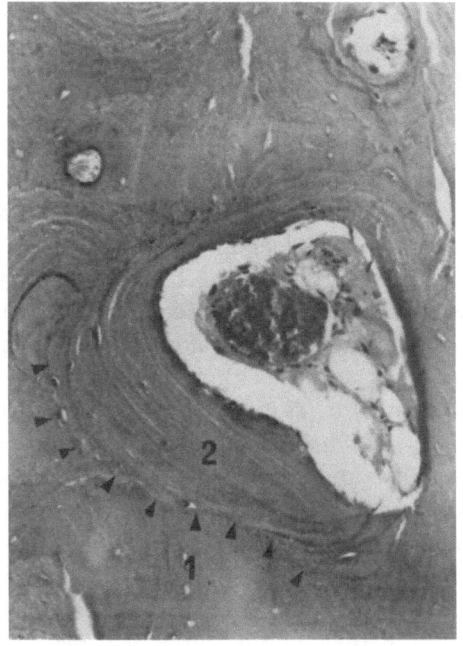

Figure VII.7 and 8. Patient 5 (B.H.S., no. 12, chapter V). The graft consists mainly of dead bone (1). Surrounding the Haversian canals, zones of living bone have been formed (2). The arrows indicate the cementing lines between dead and living bone. Figure 7, 300 ×; figure 8, 150 ×.

homogenous bone graft. The donor was a female aged 38. 1 year and 3 months later a second operation became necessary because of refracture. Bony union was found to be present between the humerus and the entire length of the graft.

Part of the humerus with the attached graft became available for histological examination.

Histologically also there was a complete fixation (fig. VII.6); it was difficult to find a plane of separation between the bone of the host and the donor graft. The part of the humerus with which the graft had united, was remarkably porotic compared with the rest of the humerus. The greater part of the graft – judged by the empty osteocyte lacunae – was dead. Adjoining the soft tissues was a zone of living bone, characterized by living osteocytes. Furthermore, throughout the entire graft, islets of living bone were found, also containing living osteocytes (fig. VII.7 and VII.8).

These islets were always situated around ingrowing bloodvessels. Practically all the Haversian canals were filled with bloodvessels, which appeared to have grown from the soft tissues as well as from the humerus. The boundary between living and dead bone was demarcated by cementing lines of irregular shape. This suggests that resorption had occurred at an earlier stage, although practically no osteoclasts were found in the specimens. In some areas of the graft there were irregularly shaped islets of immature bone. These were characterized by large osteocyte lacunae and intercellular substance of patchy basophilia. Bordering the soft tissues were well defined areas of woven bone. Massive collagenous bundles were radiating into this bone.

CONCLUSIONS

Although these data are as yet fragmentary the following preliminary conclusions about the tissue processes which follow the application of a homogenous graft may be drawn. In favourable circumstances these processes result in assimilation of the graft. The first response to the application of the graft is a stimulation of the connective tissue in the area of the wound resulting in the formation of cartilage and primitive woven bone at the surface of the graft. During the next stage of this reaction of the connective tissue we observed the penetration of vascular connective tissue via the Haversian canals of the dead graft. These vessels originate from the surrounding connective tissue as well as from the bone of the host. A similar penetration has been observed in experiments with rabbits in which autogenous or homogenous bone transplantation had been performed. The penetration of bloodvessels may give rise to different reactions. Sometimes we found a deposit of calcium compounds surrounding the bloodvessels (pathological calcification). As a rule, however, processes of remodelling take place in conjunction with the penetration of the bloodvessels: resorption is followed by bone appostion, initially of woven bone, later of lamellar bone. This remodelling takes place continuously, so that within a few years practically the entire graft has been transformed, that is to say substituted by living bone derived from the host. Owing to these processes, the graft becomes firmly attached to the bone of the host.

Thus it is the ingrowing bloodvessels which constitute the functional link between the bone of the host and the graft. Apposition of bone on the surface of the graft adjoining the receptor bone also plays a role in this fixation. In the case of patient S. there is a rarefaction of the bone structure of the humerus adjoining the graft, which has become intimately attached. This finding gives rise to the assumption that the graft has not only been taken up in the overall remodelling scheme of the humerus without any violent reactions, but that in this case it has progressed to the stage that humerus plus graft react as an entity. The graft becomes cortex which is reduced to normal proportions.

CHAPTER VIII

SUMMARY AND CONCLUSIONS

A survey is made of the bone transplantation operations performed by the authors and their colla-borators during the period from 1-2-1953 tot 1-2-1965.
958 operations are reported; in 647 fresh autogenous material was used and in 275 deep-freeze homogenous bone. The authors summarize the results, they compare the results of the homogenous transplantations with the autogenous transplantations.

The aim of this publication is to advise colleagues who would like to use homogenous bone for trans-plantation about the technique, indications and contra-indications for the use of this material.

Post-operative mortality amounted to 3 cases out of 958 operations. These were caused by sudden, massive pulmonary embolism. This low mortality shows that under the present circumstances it is possible to perform major orthopaedic operations with a wide margin of safety.
The percentage of infections in 'clean' operations was 0.6%.

A transplantation was considered to be successful if a bony union had developed between the graft and the bone tissue of the host and if the graft had been transformed into a living part of the skeletal system of the host. If this was not the case the operation was considered to be a failure. Autogenous transplantations were 86.6% successful and homogenous transplantations 87.3%.
In the chapters dealing with case histories the results are arranged and discussed according to the nature of the orthopaedic defect, and illustrated with individual case histories. For example, a total number of 269 pseudarthroses of the long bones have been treated by operation; of 195 of these cases, treated by autogenous grafting, bony union followed in 88%, of 71 cases treated by homo-genous grafting bony union followed in 87%.

The authors have reached the following conclusions regarding homogenous bone transplantation. The implantation in man of homogenous bone tissue obtained by sterile dissection and stored at low temperature, does not carry with it the danger of infection if a meticulously aseptic technique is used. The homogenous bone tissue obtained in this way does not give rise to any perceptible im-munological reactions. In several patients we have transplanted homogenous bone more than once and we have not observed any hypersensitivity reactions which could be attributed to these re-implantations. The homogenous cortical graft can be regarded as a mechanical prop; it enables the surgeon to make a solid osteosynthesis. A homogenous graft possesses the power of induction of bone formation, but only to a minor degree. The capacity of the host to reconstruct the homo-genous graft is limited in adults but is great in children.

Based on clinical, radiological and histological observations we have arrived at the following theory concerning the fate of the implanted homogenous bone graft:

– The graft is solidly fixed by the surgeon to the bone of the host if necessary with the aid of screws.
– Originating from the tissues of the host, young connective tissue develops around the graft; from this immature connective tissue bloodvessels penetrate into the graft.
– Via these ingrowing bloodvessels a remodelling of the graft takes place by the resorption and perivascular formation of new bone tissue; this penetration of bloodvessels with remodelling occurs mainly at the adjacent surfaces of the graft and bone tissue of the host, and only to a small extent in the soft tissues. The penetration of blood vessels from the bone of the host results in a bony union between this bone of the host and the graft.
– In children this remodelling is complete and the graft is completely transformed into a living part of the host's skeletal system. In adults this remodelling process is not complete; part of the graft remains and is only partly transformed into a living part of the host's skeletal system.

Because of theoretical considerations and practical experience we do not recommend the use of homogenous cancellous bone. We advise against using homogenous cancellous bone more than once in the same patient.
Our further suggestions as regards treatment, are concerned only with cortical bone graft.
Based on these suggestions we have divided the operations into 3 groups:

a. filling-up a cavity;
b. graft alongside recipient bone;
c. bridging a gap.

a. Filling-up a cavity is a good indication for using homogenous bone; cancellous bone can also be used for this purpose.

b. Placing a graft alongside bone is a comparatively good indication for using bone graft. This method is suitable for the treatment of recent fractures, pseudarthroses, some types of arthrodesis and scoliosis in children. The use of homogenous transplantation material to perform spinal fusion in *adults* must be strongly advised against.

c. A homogenous bone graft is not a suitable aid for bridging gaps in the continuity of a bone in adults. It is also not suitable for performing extra-articular arthrodesis. The homogenous graft is a useful aid in the shelf operation for congenital dysplasia of the hip.
The age of the patient is of paramount importance; the capacity for remodelling the homogenous graft is much greater in children than in adults; the application of a homogenous graft in bridging a gap in the long bones of a young child may produce splendid results in forming a complete, tubular shaft.

To these recommendations must be added the requirement that the operative technique must be beyond reproach; in performing osteosynthesis the bone bed of the host must be adequately freshened, the graft must be in close contact with the bone of the host, and the fixation must be solid.
A homogenous transplantation, in contrast to an autogenous transplantation, will not allow any surgical errors.